THE KIMCHI DIET PLAN

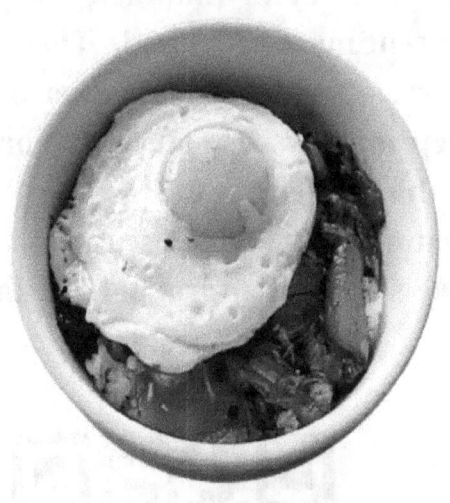

Path to Gut Health, Weight Loss, and Longevity

Anita Mark

DISCLAIMER

Acknowledgment

I would like to express my heartfelt gratitude to the rich heritage and culture of Korea, which has given birth to the art of kimjang and the diverse world of kimchi. This book would not have been possible without the generations of Korean households who have passed down their traditions, recipes, and love for kimchi.

I extend my thanks to the communities and families who have embraced the practice of kimjang, making it a cherished part of their lives and a symbol of togetherness. Your dedication to preserving this culinary heritage has inspired the pages of this book.

I would also like to acknowledge the countless individuals, both in Korea and around the world, who have shared their knowledge and passion for kimchi, enriching our understanding of this remarkable dish.

Lastly, my appreciation goes to the readers who embark on this journey with me. May the pages ahead offer you a taste of the deep-rooted history and flavors of kimchi.

Dedication

To the countless hands that have lovingly prepared kimchi throughout generations, preserving a culinary heritage and fostering a sense of community.

To the families who have gathered in the spirit of kimjang, sharing laughter and stories while creating this remarkable dish together.

To those who have embraced the art of kimchi-making as a symbol of togetherness, and to the readers who embark on this flavorful journey with us.

May this book honor your traditions, inspire your taste buds, and remind us all of the beauty in preserving cultural legacies, one batch of kimchi at a time.

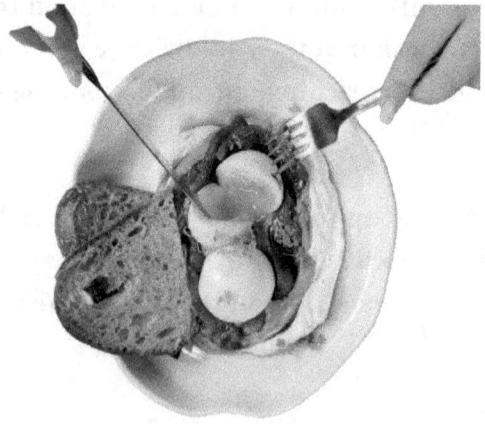

Table of Contents

Chapter 1: Kimchi History

Although no one is certain of the actual origin of kimchi, we do know that it dates back at least a few thousand years to the "Three Kingdoms" era of Korea, which lasted from 57 BCE to 668 CE. Meat, seafood, and a variety of berries, roots, and vegetables made up the early Korean cuisine. Researchers believe that the first instances of fermentation on the Korean peninsula started around this time because pots were used to store fish and vegetables between 6,000 and 3,000 BCE. Foods would have naturally fermented and been beneficial to eat because of their superior nutritional and probiotic content. Vegetables and seafood were stored carefully to safeguard them from the harsh winters and summers that were typical of the peninsula. People in Korea raised a variety of fruits, vegetables, grains including millet, rice, and later soybeans and legumes. Even before kimchi was invented, soybeans were fermented. As a result, dishes like bulgogi, which is meat marinated in fermented soybean sauce, and traditional Korean seasonings like doenjang, which is fermented soybean paste, as well as the now-famous gochujang hot paste, were created. However, the actual development of kimchi only took place between 100 BCE and 600 CE. It gained popularity as more Koreans converted to Buddhism, a faith that emphasises compassion for all living things and, as a result, a vegetarian diet.

Because specific vegetables and seasonings were more or less readily available at certain times of the year, early forms of kimchi (Kingdom Kimchi) were very different from the majority of modern recipes. Since Chinese cabbage, also known as "napa" or "kimchi" cabbage, wasn't well-liked in Korea until several hundred years later, early kimchi frequently consisted of radishes pickled in a salt paste or brine. Since red pepper (gochu) wasn't yet accessible in Korea, this particular batch of kimchi wasn't even remotely spicy. The form of kimchi that is most commonly associated with today is baechu-kimchi, which is a staple in practically every Korean household. Napak cabbage, Korean radish, gochugaru (red pepper powder), and additional flavours including garlic, ginger, and scallions are used to make it. In some cases, especially in the coastal parts of Korea, fermented seafood (jeotgal) is also added to the spice mixture.

Conflicting ideas exist on the origin of red pepper, a crucial component in the majority of modern kimchi recipes. In Japan, it is taught in schools and stated in numerous literature that red pepper was first introduced by Japan in the sixteenth century. Many Koreans dispute this claim, though, as records from Korea's Three Kingdoms period, which dates back more than 1,000 years, show that red pepper (or at least a related variety of plant) was grown for use in kimchi recipes at that time.[2] In any case, we're grateful that red pepper is now widely available throughout the world because it offers a distinctive, spicy, and warm flavour that many Koreans can't fathom living without.

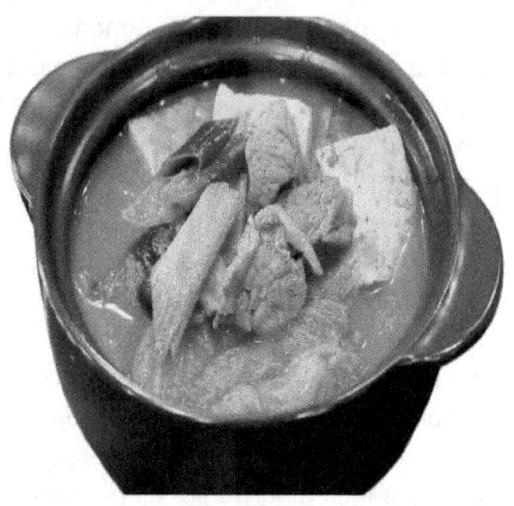

The traditional Korean supper consists of rice (bap), soup (kuk), and some type of kimchi, as well as a variety of side dishes collectively referred to as banchan. Although most Korean meals don't include kimchi, these banchan are often marinated veggies including bean sprouts, bellflower, gobo root, and radish. If they weren't vegetarians, this traditional diet allowed Koreans to consume fat and protein from animal broth and meat (typically fish) in their soups, as well as vitamins, minerals, and beneficial bacteria from kimchi, even in the cold. Additionally, the traditional Korean diet prioritises fish over red meat, includes a lot of legumes like soybeans and medicinal herbs, excludes processed and deep-fried foods, and was the first to emphasise local, seasonal ingredients and farm-to-table cooking. Korean dinners are typically served all at once, with everything on the table, giving them a truly visual feast with their variety of textures and hues. You should now be able to see why this particular diet has endured for millennia and is still practised by people all over the Korean peninsula. This should serve as motivation for our own dietary choices wherever we may reside.

Kimjang & Local Kimchi Varieties

The practise of producing kimchi has its roots in the above-mentioned tradition of kimjang, which is a one-month period in part of November and December when tens of thousands of households throughout Korea prepare their excess from the fall crop for storage throughout the winter. Kimchi was one of the only foodstuffs that provided the ancient Koreans with the critical vitamins and minerals they needed during the colder seasons when veggies were scarce. But the requisite actions for kimjang start months beforehand. Seafood was usually bought in the spring. Vegetables matured for harvest in the autumn, and sea salt was purchased throughout the summer. Kimjang demanded that the entire society participate, just as every member of the family did. The husband would have to pay for the vegetables that his family didn't grow themselves, such as scallions, radishes, garlic, fish, and ginger. Wives handled all aspects of food preparation, including cleaning, cutting, salting, and winterizing the veggies. Throughout the winter, kimchi was traditionally kept underground in earthenware clay storage pots. The community as a whole was involved in the process, not just individual households. They would collaborate, celebrate, and frequently share different kinds of kimchi with their friends and family. Based on varying fermentation times, levels of saltiness and spice, and of course, the veggies utilised, each region and even each village would make a different sort of kimchi.

As a result, each region in Korea has earned a reputation for particular varieties of kimchi that endure to this day. Jeotgal, a less salted seafood, is used in Gangwon-do, whereas squid, flatfish, and pollock are used in Hamgyeong-do, to the north. In comparison to its neighbour Hwanghae-do, Pyeongan-do is recognised for milder, more watery kimchis. Hwanghae-do also has a more neutral flavour because it doesn't contain the red pepper powder common to most kimchi sold in supermarkets. As is the case with its neighbour to the west, Jeolla-do, which incorporates fermented fish and red pepper, Gyeongsang-so in the southeast boasts some of the saltiest and spicier kimchi. It's really a destination for individuals who enjoy extremes.

With more than 250 varieties of kimchi, each region of Korea is renowned for its unique cuisine, just as in the United States, people may debate the merits of deep-dish Chicago pizza versus New York pizza as well as the use of completely different toppings like pineapple, sun dried tomatoes, or barbecued chicken! These regional distinctions have some value lost after World War II and the advent of mass production. However, traditional methods of preparing kimchi do not vanish suddenly. Particularly true of rural residents who continue to prepare kimchi in the traditional manner are the areas' distinctive methods of preparing, salting, and seasoning the dish.

A Variety of Kimchi

Which of the 250 varieties of kimchi that Korea has created throughout the years are some of the most popular? First off, most people probably associate kimchi with the hot, fermented dish made from napa cabbage known as baechu-kimchi, but there are many more kimchi recipes that aren't hot and don't even include cabbage. In truth, baechu-kimchi may be a much more recent contribution to the Korean cuisine than napa cabbage, having previously been prepared with radishes, open-leaved cabbages, scallions, fish, and even grains.

As previously said, historically, the vegetables and seasonings used in kimchi recipes have been greatly influenced by what is in season in each region of Korea. Seafood that has been fermented and salted, such as prawns, fish, clams and oysters, is known as "jeotgal" and is frequently used as a flavouring in coastal areas.

Depending on what could be grown locally each season in the more inland areas, different veggies and seasonings were employed.

Kimchi is frequently believed to be always fermenting. It's also frequently eaten fresh, especially in the summer, even though fermenting it for a few days to a few months may make it more flavorful and addicting. Baechu-geotjeori, a type of fresh unfermented kimchi prepared using cabbage, is another option. Fresh kimchi can also be created with other vegetables, such as cucumbers and Korean radishes.

Right before winter officially begins, dongchimi (radish water kimchi) is typically made using fresh radishes and fermented with the traditional kimchi ingredients. Although everyone has a distinct favourite, I enjoy both dongchimi and cabbage kimchi equally despite the fact that they have very different flavours and textures. My dongchimi recipe can be found in the Resources section.

Using persimmons, radish, and cabbage, gam kimchi is made. So yes, you can make kimchi out of fruit! For those who enjoy Halloween, you'll be happy to know that pumpkins can be used to make a type of kimchi called hobak kimchi.

Oi kimchi, which I believe practically everyone who has never tried kimchi would adore, is another favourite. When starting The Kimchi DietTM, I advise everyone to start with this particular kimchi because it is made with cucumbers rather than napa cabbage or radishes. Oi kimchi, which may be consumed both fresh and fermented, is a deliciously cooling summertime kimchi.

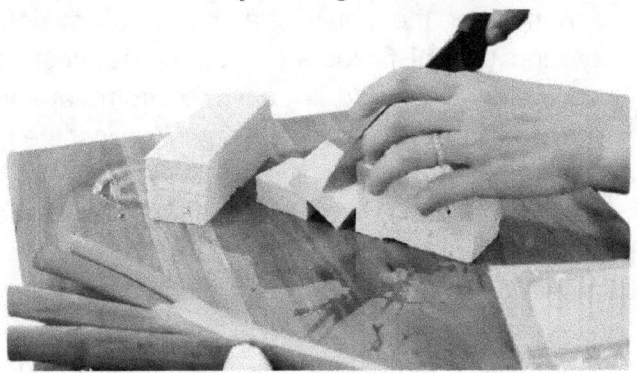

Summertime is a popular time to prepare and consume nabak kimchi, also known as water kimchi. Compared to other kimchi recipes, it has a lot more brine, which is salty. The savoury broth can be used to make soup, used as a topping for rice or noodles, or just sipped on its own to soothe one's thirst. These less complicated kimchis were frequently prepared in the summertime and required less work than those prepared in the chilly kimjang winters.

To get you started on the right track to better health, I've included my Kimchi DietTM Recipes for each phase of the programme in Chapter 5 of this book, including the cucumber kimchi recipe.

Today's Kimchi

Today, eating kimchi is a delicious and satisfying experience for the palate that combines sweet, sour, salty, and umami flavours (umami is the most recently discovered flavour and is translated from Japanese as savoury and tasty). Basically, "kimchi" is just the Korean name for "fermented vegetables." Nowadays, napa cabbage or radishes are typically fermented to create it. But practically any kind of vegetable and some fruits can be used to make it. Red peppers and other ingredients can be used in its preparation.

The probiotics, the beneficial intestinal bacteria found in fermented foods like yoghurt, sauerkraut, and kefir, give it a particular health-giving one-two punch of super nutritious veggies and magical abilities. We'll explore its numerous health advantages in more detail in Chapter 2.

In the last century, kimchi's fame has grown immensely, and it is currently widely consumed in many nations around the world. Koreans consume 40 to 50 pounds of kimchi on average per year, with 63% of it still being prepared at home.[3] Numerous neighbouring nations either purchase kimchi from Korea or produce their own, including for export. In contrast, a large portion of the kimchi consumed in Korea is now produced at a low cost in China as a result of industrialization and mass manufacturing, with Japan accounting for about 80% of Korea's kimchi exports. I like kimchi prepared in Korea since it typically tastes better and isn't made with chemicals or food additives. Kimchi is available in most Asian markets, health food shops, and even some regular supermarkets in the United States. However, even in many ostensibly "healthy" kimchi packets, additives and chemicals should be avoided.

It's terrible because fermented foods are still a fantastic way to preserve food for extended periods of time without the need for refrigeration. Prior to the industrial revolution, fermented foods were far more widely consumed than they are now. Regarding nutrition and their advantageous impacts on gut health, they are hard to top. But with the development of refrigeration, veggies may now be preserved for a longer period of time. Unfavourable side effect: Prior to the widespread adoption of refrigeration, humans had to devise the best methods for preserving food for as long as possible. The most common method for carrying out this activity has traditionally been fermentation. This method of food preservation was utilised to preserve bread, alcohol, fruits, vegetables, dairy products, and pretty much every other sort of food imaginable. It also had a number of health advantages that a refrigerator can't match.

Many people from all over the world, including many Koreans, prefer to purchase kimchi and other fermented dishes from the grocery store rather than creating their own in today's busy world where convenience is king. MSG and other artificial sweeteners and chemicals are frequently added to store-bought variations. But as long as it's all-natural, unpasteurized, and as close to homemade kimchi as possible, eating store-bought kimchi can still provide a variety of nutritional benefits.

Fermentation Methods

Fermenting various foods and beverages has been practised for thousands of years around the world. From clay pots to sophisticated airtight containers, each civilization has created its own distinctive methods of manufacturing and conserving its valuable items. If you're unfamiliar with the fermentation process, here's a quick primer.

Food fermentation is a natural process that occurs in an anaerobic (oxygen-free) environment, in which yeasts and bacteria (including multiple strains of lactic acid bacteria, or LAB) that are naturally present on the food convert starches and sugars into various acids and alcohols. To prevent dangerous moulds and undesired germs from forming, vegetables are typically fermented in a salt brine (salt and water mixture) or a salty paste. Although salt causes lactic acid bacteria to grow and spread, it also destroys almost all dangerous bacteria in fermented foods, such as E. Coli. Good bacteria feed on the vegetables (and other foods used), releasing acids and gases that help us preserve the food. We acquire tremendous nourishment and these beneficial lactic acid bacteria when we eat the meal.

Fermentation can take anywhere from a few days to many months, depending on the type of fermented food, the ambient temperature, and how ripe or sour you wish it to taste. Once properly fermented, the meal is normally stored in a cool place, such as the refrigerator, a cellar, or in the ground (depending on the season and location). This significantly slows down the fermentation process, allowing you to enjoy the dish before it becomes too sour or mushy. Many civilizations have traditionally fermented vegetables in order to have a supply for the winter months. Instead of wasting the surplus of the autumn crop, humans devised a clever way to eat vegetables throughout the cold months of December, January, and February (in the northern hemisphere). They not only prevented spoilage, but they also developed some of the world's first superfoods, which were high in probiotic microorganisms. These "friendly" bacteria are extremely beneficial in maintaining healthy digestion, immunological function, and a variety of other functions.

Even before we realised they existed, humans had a long and deep relationship with the bacteria present in our food. For ages, we've fermented food to increase the shelf life of our crop, to make food more pleasant (certain foods, such as cabbage, taste far better fermented than raw), and because we've discovered some foods to have high nutritional and medicinal value.

World Fermented Foods

Korea's most prominent contribution to the world of fermented cuisine is flavorful kimchi, but the country is also recognised for fermented soybean paste and soy sauce (which originated in Korea), fermented red pepper powder paste, and fermented fish, to name a few more delectable concoctions. While this book concentrates on kimchi, I wanted to discuss some of the other foods you might want to try if you want to get the most out of the world's fermented meals and the beneficial bacteria contained in them.

Yoghurt

Yoghurt is the most popular cultured food in the United States, and it is likely that most individuals eat it on a regular basis. Despite the lack of definitive evidence, many scientists believe yoghurt was originated in the Middle East around 7,000 years ago. There are now dozens of yoghurt flavours available, ranging from blueberry and strawberry to Greek yoghurt and dairy-free coconut yoghurt. Unfortunately, typical milk-based yoghurt is one of the fermented foods that I am least likely to offer to anyone seeking my nutritional guidance. The truth is that most yoghurt sold in supermarkets is made with pasteurised milk, which might reduce the amount of beneficial bacteria you consume. Furthermore, it frequently has a high concentration of sugar and other chemicals, resulting in low lactic acid bacteria numbers. Companies are ruining the health benefits of traditional yoghurt by reintroducing sugar or phoney additives. This is true even for many ostensibly "healthy" yoghurts, such as those made with nondairy milks. Aside from this proclivity for extra sweets, yoghurt creates digestive issues for many people. Many people are intolerant or sensitive to dairy, many of whom are unaware. They may have excessive bloating, gas, constipation, or diarrhoea. Some people acquire skin problems like acne or eczema. Personally, I recommend almond, coconut, or rice milk yoghurts. Also, ensure that they have not been pasteurised. If you take this way, coconut or almond yoghurt are probably the best choices.

Pickles

Pickles are prepared from cucumbers fermented in a salty brine (often with garlic or other flavours added) and are the second most common fermented food consumed in the United States. They're crunchy, acidic, and refreshing, and Kosher Dills, which are now widely available in stores, have been relished for generations by Jewish people in Eastern Europe. When immigrants from this region immigrated to the United States, they brought their pickling practises with them, establishing pickles as a staple on a variety of sandwiches and burgers.

Pickles are a quick and easy way to preserve an overflow of cucumbers that you might have at the end of summer if you have a vegetable garden. Unfortunately, most pickles in grocery stores these days have been pasteurised, which means they've lost their probiotics and living enzymes. Or they've been preserved in vinegar rather than pickled in salt brine. However, fermenting and preserving your own pickles is a terrific practise that will help you to reap the full health advantages of the lactic acid bacteria found in them. Cucumber kimchi, made from cut-up cucumbers, is light and delicious for the summer and is frequently made without fiery red pepper.

Bread with Sourdough

Another popular bread around the world is sourdough, which is thought to have originated in ancient Egypt thousands of years ago. Sourdough was the way for leavening breads of all kinds before baker's yeast was invented in the last century, and this ancient process is being used today all over the world. Sourdough bread has more nutrients, is easier to digest, and has a richer flavour than bread produced with commercial yeast. Similarly to pickles, European immigrants to America in the 1800s brought their prized sourdough starter culture with them on the long boat voyage over. That is devotion!

Unfortunately, most wheat farmed in the United States contains GMOs (genetically modified organisms) and has been heavily sprayed with the harmful glyphosate. Glyphosate use has been connected to gluten intolerance and sensitivity, and many gluten intolerant or sensitive people see significant improvement when they quit eating bread--even sourdough. Others who are not gluten intolerant simply experience the negative effects of these substances and feel better when they consume organic wheat. In my three decades of working with nutrition, however, I've seen significant improvements in the health of almost everyone I've encouraged to stop eating gluten, as it's difficult for the body to process and can cause gas, bloating, irritable bowel syndrome, brain fog, lethargy, and a slew of other symptoms. Because of these considerations, the advantages of sourdough just exceed the disadvantages of gluten consumption, and you're better off sticking to your own pickled vegetables, plant-based yoghurts, and, of course, kimchi! I don't recommend eating sourdough or any other wheat-based product unless you're convinced it won't cause you any problems.

Sauerkraut

Sauerkraut, a fermented cabbage meal said to have originated in Germany, is another fermented cuisine you're definitely familiar with. It's prepared in the same way that Kimchi is, by fermenting shredded cabbage in a salt water brine (made with table salt or sea salt and water). It's really simple to prepare at home, tastes acidic and slightly sweet, and begins with a lovely crunch. The cabbage will become softer and softer over time. It's popular on sandwiches and as a side dish. Today, you can get sauerkraut in almost any grocery store, but much of it has been pasteurised, removing many of its nutrients as well as all of its probiotics. The lesson is straightforward: handmade is superior. For the greatest health advantages, choose raw, unpasteurized fermented veggies (ideally organic). Because of its nutritional profile and other elements, sauerkraut is perhaps the best fermented food, second only to kimchi

Kvass with Kefir

Milk kefir and kvass, both of which originated in Russia, are two popular non-alcoholic fermented beverages. Kefir is a fermented dairy drink produced from cow, goat, or sheep milk. After a few days of fermentation at room temperature, it thickens slightly but remains palatable and pourable. Kvass was historically produced from fermented rye or other naturally leavened bread in water, but it is now also made with beets and other fruits and vegetables. If you want to drink kefir, look for plant-based varieties. Homemade kvass with beets can also be delicious--just avoid using bread if you're gluten-intolerant.

Kombucha

While kombucha may appear to be a healthy alternative, I've seen many patients who drink it on a regular basis develop extra yeast and bacterial overgrowth in their stomach. My clinical practise has validated this with lab stool tests. Excess yeast and bacteria can cause SIBO (small intestine bacterial overgrowth) and SIFO (small intestine fungal overgrowth), which puts the microbiome out of balance. Kombucha contains alcohol as well as a lot of sugar. As a result, I recommend avoiding kombucha.

These are just a few examples of fermented foods and beverages that have been staples of the human diet for thousands of years and will hopefully continue to be for many thousands more.

Kimchi: The All-Powerful Superfood

So, what distinguishes kimchi from the dozens of other fermented foods? Why is it a superfood that is not only comparable to, but even superior to, yoghurt, sourdough, kefir, and sauerkraut?

The first thing to observe is that kimchi combines numerous components, so you get all of the vitamins and nutrients from everything in the combination. Whereas sauerkraut provides the health advantages of cabbage, kimchi is the outcome of collaboration. When you eat traditional baechu-kimchi, you are getting the advantages of napa cabbage as well as radishes, green onions, garlic, ginger, red pepper powder, shellfish, and other components. Let's break it down and look at the health advantages of each element individually.

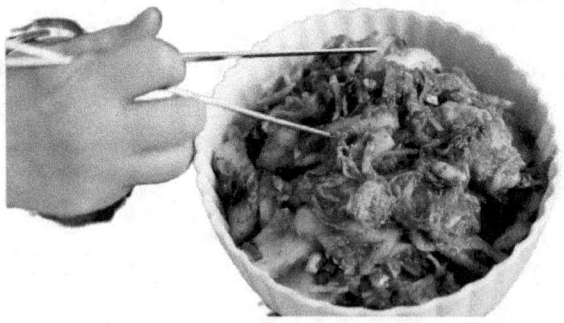

We'll look at the most well-known kimchi, baechu-kimchi. Vitamin C and carotene, which the body converts to vitamin A, are found in napa cabbage. Radishes are also high in vitamin C and minerals like calcium and phosphorus, which aid with bone development.

Red peppers are high in vitamins and one of the primary reasons that dangerous bacteria do not develop in kimchi while beneficial bacteria flourish. Jeotgal, fermented fish, adds flavour as well as important amino acids that can help improve the immune system, develop muscle, and do other things. However, it is not required, and vegan kimchi can be created.

Garlic has significant concentrations of allicin, which "binds to harmful substances in the human body and allows them to be discharged, thereby detoxifying the body of heavy metals and other such harmful substances."[4] Spring onions, like garlic, contain allicin, which can help prevent hazardous germs from forming in the fermented mixture.

As you can see, no other fermented meal on the planet that is based solely on single components can compete with this combination of vitamins, minerals, and amino acids. Don't forget that you may replace pumpkins, persimmons, or a variety of other veggies for napa cabbage and reap the health benefits of those meals all year.

The second advantage of kimchi is that it is low in calories, all-natural, and largely plant-based, making it more full. Prior to the growth of industrialization in the 1960s and 1970s, Koreans did not face nearly the same level of modern epidemics such as heart disease, obesity, and high blood pressure. Even now, their numbers are minimal in comparison to Americans. Remember that most Koreans ate some sort of kimchi at practically every meal in the past, and this practise continues to this day.

According to some estimations, the average daily consumption of kimchi has decreased from roughly 300 grammes to 60-100 grammes today.[5] That is, traditionally, Koreans would eat vegetables throughout the day, filling up on fiber-rich kimchi loaded with billions of probiotic organisms, rather than eating potentially unhealthy foods like burgers, pizza, bagels, and pasta, which are so prevalent in the standard American diet. The average serving of kimchi (one cup) contains 45-90 calories.

If we use the low value of 45 calories, that equates to around four potato chips. Consider how quickly a plate of kimchi can fill you up versus four chips! Even one cup of yoghurt has 100 calories and is unlikely to satisfy you as much as a plate of kimchi. It's no surprise that Koreans were able to fill up on delicious delicacies while maintaining a healthy weight by eating plenty of cabbage, radish, and other veggies.

The third advantage of kimchi is similar to that of other fermented foods: the production of lactic acid bacteria and other probiotics during the fermenting process. Probiotics have been related to a slew of health advantages, which will be covered in Chapter 2. But, in a nutshell, our intestinal tract is teeming with billions of bacteria, many of which are beneficial and others of which are toxic. Through the vagus nerve, which connects to the brain, these bacteria aid in everything from digestion to energy production to mood management. The more harmful bacteria, pathogenic yeasts, parasites, and viruses proliferate in our stomach, the worse our health can get. Microbial imbalances can cause bloating, digestive difficulties, inflammation, and even anxiety and melancholy. We absorb millions of different strains of helpful bacteria when we eat kimchi. In fact, over 2,300 lactic acid bacteria strains have been discovered in kimchi! Compare this to the five or so strains provided by most probiotic tablets. You just cannot compete with naturally fermented foods. You also receive all of the advantages of eating real, entire, raw, and living foods.

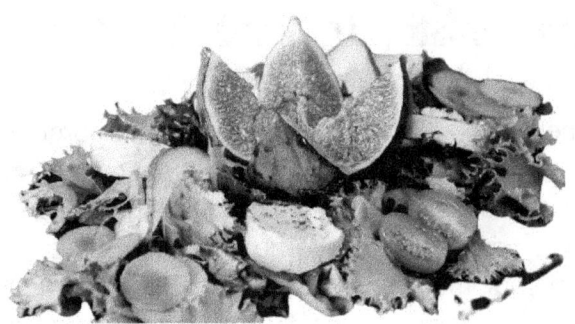

Chapter 2: The Science and Health Benefits of Kimchi

Kimchi is one of the world's healthiest foods. Everyone knows that vegetables, especially leafy greens like napa cabbage, which makes up the majority of kimchi recipes, are extremely healthful on their own. However, when changed by lactic acid bacteria through the magical process of fermentation, modest vegetables become something even better, capable of boosting and preserving our health even more than the vegetables in their natural state.

Kimchi is naturally cholesterol-free (if veganized), low in fat and calories, and high in fibre, vitamins, minerals, and phytochemicals. It also has all of the nutritious benefits of ginger, garlic, red peppers, scallions, and any other vegetables you choose--all in one. We'll go over some of the advantages of these additional substances further down.

The Fantastic Human Microbiome

Most Americans have probably heard about probiotics and the importance of having good gut bacteria by now. The universe of microorganisms that reside in each of our bodies, primarily in our large intestine, is known as our gut microbiome. These bacteria total more than 100 trillion and can weigh up to five pounds! A disturbing figure that made the rounds online was that humans had 10 times as many bacterial cells in our body as human cells, but newer research suggests that the ratio may be closer to a 1:1 ratio. In any case, we're just as much "bacteria" as we are "human." So, doesn't it make sense to do everything we can to encourage the growth of helpful bacteria while eradicating harmful ones? Kimchi's power is once again unrivalled!

However, investigating the gut microbiome remains one of the most cutting-edge areas of scientific inquiry, with scientists only now beginning to understand all of the roles that these bacteria play in our biological processes. Although one of the world's first microbiologists, Antonie van Leeuwenhoek, began studying the human microbiome at least several hundred years ago, it was ignored as scientists instead focused on organ systems, brain function, and macrological features of the human body. The microorganisms in the human body captivated the Dutch scientist van Leeuwenhoek, now regarded as "The Father of Microbiology," as he was one of the first to see them. He described these microorganisms as follows: "I then most always saw, with great wonder, that in the said matter there were many very little living animalcules, very prettily a-moving."

Since van Leeuwenhoek's time, we've learnt a lot, and in recent decades, experts all around the world have dedicated their lives to studying the human microbiome.

They're tasked with sequencing a nearly endless number of bacterial, viral, fungal, and protozoa strains found in our bodies. They're also trying to figure out how these microbes affect human health and body functioning. So far, there are really strong signs that our microbiome is crucial to our health and that the bacteria and other species that live in our gut actually help us a lot.

Our mitochondria, the cells' powerhouses, are ancient prokaryotes. These developed bacteria collaborated with nearly every cell in our body to offer us with energy in exchange for protection from the elements. They currently account for roughly 10% of our total body mass. Consider how essential germs are to human survival!

So what exactly do gut microbes do? We're only now beginning to grasp their numerous jobs, but it's apparent that when we have too many of the incorrect sorts of bacteria in our gut, or not enough of the healthy ones, mayhem ensues in the shape of everything from weight problems to digestive troubles to allergies. We also know that beneficial gut bacteria help our bodies by battling bad bacteria, digesting carbohydrates, reducing inflammation, and strengthening our immune system.

According to Harvard Medical School, there is "some evidence that a specific strain of the bacterium Lactobacillus johnsonii may protect against some cancers," and another study found that the bacteria strain "Akkermansia muciniphila" could prevent inflammation that contributes to fatty plaque buildup in arteries, which is a leading cause of heart disease.[2] Other research has connected an excess of pathogenic gut bacteria to "chronic diseases like inflammatory bowel disease, obesity, cancer, and autism."[3] These studies have brought the role of probiotics--bacteria that are good to human function--to the forefront. Probiotic content in kombucha, yoghurt, and sauerkraut is eagerly advertised by food makers, and individuals spend billions of dollars each year on probiotic supplements. I don't recommend drinking kombucha in particular because of the risk of yeast and bacterial overgrowth, as well as the high sugar and alcohol content.

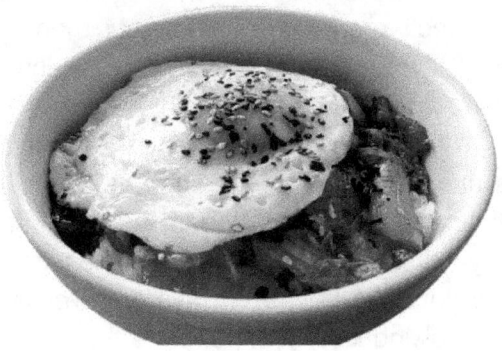

Probiotic probiotics in capsule form have been used by early adopters for a decade or more. What they may not realise is that eating raw, fermented foods is both less expensive and more effective than taking probiotic pills. A single jar of kimchi or sauerkraut contains the same number of probiotic bacteria as eight to ten bottles of probiotic pills! And the components for that single jar of kimchi or sauerkraut aren't much more than a few dollars.

Changing what we eat has been demonstrated in study after research to be one of the quickest and most effective strategies to transform our gut flora. Babies fed breast milk or traditional formulas have different amounts of the predominant gut bacteria, and "short-term consumption of diets composed entirely of animal meat, eggs, and cheeses or plant-rich in grains, fruits, legumes, and vegetables altered microbial community structure and overwhelmed inter-individual differences in microbial gene expression."[4] That is, the effects of their meals, whether protein based or plant-based,were more relevant than any inborn bacterial differences in individuals. This isn't to imply we shouldn't eat nutritious proteins like fish or grass-fed beef. It does, however, imply that including more plant foods and fermented foods such as kimchi can make a significant difference in modifying our internal biome. What you'll discover in this book has the potential to change your gut biome in days and weeks, rather than years, allowing you to experience the health benefits of kimchi that Koreans have known about for millennia.

Why Do Kimchi Ingredients Matter?

Organic foods have been proved to have numerous health benefits throughout the years, but more research is needed to determine the entire range of advantages organic foods have over conventionally cultivated products. Many health advantages, on the other hand, have been well proven. Some chemicals, such as glyphosate, the world's most widely used herbicide, are classified as "probable carcinogens" by the World Health Organisation, despite the fact that this chemical is frequently sprayed all over conventionally cultivated wheat fields and other crops. Roundup®, in particular, has come under fire for its potentially hazardous effects.[5] This is reason enough to buy organic produce whenever feasible.

Organic vegetables may also be more nutritious than conventionally farmed vegetables. A six-year study of onions found that organic onions have 20% more antioxidants than conventionally cultivated onions.[6] Remember that antioxidants are in charge of combating "free radicals," which are unstable chemicals that connect fast to parts of the body and cause cellular deterioration. Radiation, cigarette smoke, narcotics, and pesticides are all sources of free radicals. These free radicals generate oxidative stress, which results in a "rusting" effect in the body and can play a role in a variety of disorders, including:

Heart Disease and Cancer

Lumpus

Alzheimer's

Arthritis

Free radicals are also thought to contribute to premature ageing since they wear down the body over time if not "captured" and dealt with by antioxidants. You may obtain more antioxidants from organic foods, including the organic vegetables in kimchi, which is one of their key health benefits. By avoiding pesticides, you are reducing your exposure to free radicals.

As a result, it's very crucial to use organic ingredients in all of your kimchi recipes. While more people are coming to realise the health advantages of organic foods in general, recent study has been conducted specifically on the impact of organic meals on kimchi and probiotic production. According to the study "Physiochemical and Quality Characteristics of Young Radish (Yulmoo) Kimchi Cultivated by Organic Farming" (2014), organic radishes outperformed control groups of conventionally grown radishes in terms of producing more helpful bacteria and increasing the freshness and nutritional content of kimchi.[8] Unsurprisingly, beneficial bacteria thrive on food that has not been sprayed with pesticides and chemicals designed to kill or repel diverse life forms. Not only that, but participants in the study thought the organic kimchi was more visually appealing! You may maximise the nutritional potential of homemade kimchi and make it gentler on the body by using organic cabbage, radishes, peppers, and other components.

It's also vital to consider the type of salt you use. While it may not appear to be a significant concern, using the wrong salt can alter the taste, appearance, and overall outcome of your kimchi. In a study conducted in Korea, different salt kinds were examined for both acidity levels and how participants reacted to each after a tasting test.[10] Purified salt, which is most commonly found in shops and restaurants, was compared to sea salt for the purposes of the study. The researchers discovered that using refined salt increased acid levels faster and made the kimchi soggier faster. In contrast, sea salt kept the kimchi crisper, and the acid levels rose gradually. Iodized refined table salt can potentially be a problem. Participants once again favoured kimchi made with sea salt over kimchi made with purified salt.[11] However, not all sea salts are created equal. Himalayan salt contains approximately 95% sodium chloride with low mineral levels, whereas other salts may contain only 70% sodium chloride with greater quantities of calcium, magnesium, and phosphorus. sun sea salt, particularly Korean or Celtic sun sea salt, is ideal.

Kimchi Fermentation Method

So, how does kimchi ferment, and what effect does this magical process have on the beneficial components of the cabbages, radishes, garlic, ginger, and/or peppers that you bite into weeks later? At its most basic, fermentation is the process by which bacteria break down the carbohydrates in food in order to sustain themselves anaerobically (without oxygen). They emit alcohols, fumes, or acid as a result of this process. Beer, wine, spirits, or Korea's favourite, soju, are produced when they exhale alcohol. When we ferment foods, we encourage the growth of specific types of bacteria. Temperature, pH, oxygen levels, and fermentation time all influence how rapidly or slowly these bacteria grow.

If you've done it correctly, these bacteria will eventually outnumber and outcompete the microorganisms that would ordinarily result in food decomposition and putrefaction, and the bacteria, together with brining, will assist to preserve the kimchi for longer. Probiotic bacteria develop on kimchi, and these helpful bacteria are important for our gut, immune system, digestion, and more. Kimchi is home to a variety of bacteria, with representatives of the species Leuconostoc, Lactobacillus, and Weissella dominating at different stages of fermentation.[12] And each of these microorganisms has numerous health benefits for your body. Lactobacillus, for example, may lower cholesterol, combat colds and flus, aid in weight loss, and alleviate allergies and eczema, in addition to boosting general gut health.[13] To speed up the process, lactic acid bacteria starters can be utilised, albeit this is mostly used in commercial kimchi manufacturing. Kimchi does not require a starter because the lactic acid bacteria on your hands and the vegetables are plenty! If you have any skin disorders, such as eczema, psoriasis, or fungal infections, it's better to wear gloves to avoid disrupting the fermentation process.

The primary criticism about over-fermentation is what it does to the taste. Allowing the kimchi to develop for too long can result in an increasingly sour or acidic flavour due to the buildup of chemicals released by the bacteria. However, improper fermentation methods in commercial production have been linked to E.coli and norovirus outbreaks, though these are extremely rare because the probiotics in kimchi do such a good job of attacking and overpowering any harmful bacteria that may grow on the kimchi due to contamination. Still, this is another reason to cook it at home. Kimchi, because to its pH and lactic acid bacteria composition, is exceptionally safe, killing off most dangerous bacteria and organisms.

Kimchi's Health Benefits

There are virtually endless possible health benefits of eating kimchi on a regular basis. Most of these advantages are supported by research, which I will address further below. Other advantages, which are not addressed here because they have not been scientifically validated, have been passed down as sacred knowledge through many generations in Korea and abroad. Every day, scientists confirm more and more of what Koreans instinctively know about how amazing kimchi tastes, and I wouldn't be surprised to see a growing quantity of literature justify this traditional wisdom as the years pass.

These are just a few of the many scientifically proven benefits of including kimchi into your diet:

- Better Immunity and Gut Health

- Improved Digestion and Elimination

- Weight Loss and Body Contouring

- Cardiovascular Health

- Anti-Aging and Antioxidant Properties

- More Power

- Skin That Is Clearer and More Vibrant

- Mood Enhancer

- Increased Mental Clarity

- Healthy Blood Pressure

- Anti-Mutagenic and Cancer Prevention

Let's take a closer look at each of these life-changing benefits to better grasp kimchi's ability to alter your health.

SIBO, Gut Health, and Immunity

Eating kimchi is one of the best things you can do to boost your immune system. Aside from being high in vitamin C, kimchi contains probiotics such as lactic acid bacteria, which are also found in yoghurt. Simply put, when healthy bacteria outnumber and dominate bad bacteria, yeasts, and parasites--including those that cause illness or impair immune function--we feel better.

Most individuals are unaware that our gut contains 70-80% of our immune system. This is known as the Gut Associated Lymphoid Tissue (GALT). It's where the battle between probiotics and dangerous bacteria and viruses--the ones that cause colds and flus--most frequently takes place. Our gut is sometimes referred to as our second brain, and for good reason: it is extremely intelligent when it comes to battling sickness! Many of our neurotransmitters and immune-fighting substances, such as antibodies, are created by cells in our small intestine, our body's longest organ.
[14] The strength of billions of live probiotic bacteria found in each serving of kimchi, along with an

astonishing array of vitamins, minerals, and many phytonutrients, makes it a strong contender against any wayward virus, bacterium, or fungi that may try to wreak havoc in your body. According to one study, one of the most common species of lactic acid bacteria in kimchi, L. Mesenteroides, produces cyclic dipeptides with antibacterial activity (Liu et al. 2017).[15] And, as we'll see later, a stronger immune system with fewer germs attacking it is much better able to avoid catastrophic health problems like cancer.

Our gut microbiota is also responsible for numerous critical immune-related processes. Our moms pass on to us our gut biome and the types of bacteria we inherit at birth. As a result, the relative health of your mother's gut flora can influence yours at a young age. Similarly, for female readers, what you eat now can assist enhance the microbiome of any children you may have in the future. As Broussard and Devkota have demonstrated, a wide range of modern epidemics, from diabetes to irritable bowel syndrome (IBS) to allergies and more, may be traceable to the difference between the types of bacteria humans used to have and the new types of gut biomes that arose as a result of industrialised food production and modern lifestyles.[16] In other words, we've changed our gut biomes through time and inherited new bacteria from our mothers, not all of which are good for processing nutrients and fighting disease. The authors explain, in particular, how easy access to refined sugars and simple carbs has become a major element of the Western diet, and how the shift away from fiber-rich foods permits unhealthy gut biomes to flourish. The scientists make the following observations:

Human research comparing metabolic disease incidence in Western versus non-Western food patterns can provide additional insights. Diabetes and obesity are almost unheard of in these native cultures, regardless of geographic location.[17]

Again, the presence of bacteria more similar to those seen in our ancestors' diets--focused on local, organic, fiber-rich, unprocessed foods--seems to help people thrive. The healthier the gut flora and diversity, it appears, the lower the risk of diabetes and obesity. Kimchi is a clear winner in terms of its capacity to be created naturally, its probiotic content, and its fibre content!

But there's more. Excess carbohydrate and sugar consumption in some people can result in an overgrowth of bacteria in the small intestine, known as SIBO (small intestinal bacterial overgrowth), because the bacteria feed on sugars. SIBO has just recently become recognised as a more common diagnosis--the outcome of an overabundance of microorganisms. It has been connected to irritable bowel syndrome by Dukowicz, Lacy, and Levine (2014), as well as "frequently implicated as the cause of chronic diarrhoea and malabsorption." Patients with SIBO may also experience inadvertent weight loss, nutritional deficits, and osteoporosis."[18] SIBO, on the other hand, has been linked to a slew of more serious illnesses. One study discovered a strong link between restless leg syndrome and SIBO, as well as irritable bowel syndrome.[19] In a 2015 study, a quarter of patients with unexplained GI symptoms like bloating, gas, and nausea were found to have SIFO (Small Intestinal Fungal Overgrowth), often known as Candidiasis.[20] But the consequences of SIBO are far-reaching. SIBO was discovered in a considerable number (44%) of Type 1 Diabetics with autonomic neuropathy. The study discovered that those patients had a higher daily insulin demand than Type 1 diabetics without autonomic neuropathy.[21] If this describes you, introducing kimchi into your diet, combined with a proportional reduction in your sugar intake, can be beneficial. The less sugar you consume, the less hazardous fungus and bacteria develop. And the more probiotic-rich foods you consume, such as kimchi, the more the lactic acid bacteria can aid in the fight against the evil guys.

Finally, in a 2016 study of Chinese patients with MS (Multiple Sclerosis), 38% tested positive for SIBO, compared to 8% in the control group.[22] Again, the causal relationship is unclear, but there appears to be a link between bacterial overgrowth and a variety of health concerns. More research is needed to discover the specific link, but the good news is eating kimchi can help to alleviate both issues.

There's another reason why kimchi is so important for our gut health, particularly in terms of immunity. We've reached a stage in our medical system when antibiotics have lost most of their potency due to overuse, culminating in the emergence of "superbugs," harmful bacteria that are now extraordinarily resistant to antibiotics as they evolve over time. Instead of being easily treated with antibiotics, these superbugs are free to spread and grow. Unfortunately, this implies that people are dying from diseases that were once easily treated with a prescription for an antibiotic. Each year, more than two million people in the United States become sick with antibiotic-resistant bacteria, and over 23,000 of them die as a result of these infections.

Can the Diarrhoea Ever Stop?

Robert, a forty-nine-year-old male CEO, had a severe bout of diarrhoea. He would use the restroom 10-12 times each day, dealing with everything from loose stools to watery, projectile diarrhoea. His symptoms began six months before he saw me, following three rounds of antibiotics for a chronic sinus infection. The same doctor who ordered the antibiotics suggested Robert use an over-the-counter pink liquid to stop the diarrhoea since he might have an irritated intestine due to his stressful job. He came into my office irritated and fatigued with his illness, and he wanted to find out what was causing his diarrhoea.

I perform a stool analysis on all of my diarrhoea patients to screen for pathogenic bacteria and parasites, and the findings were positive for a Clostridium difficile (C. diff) infection.

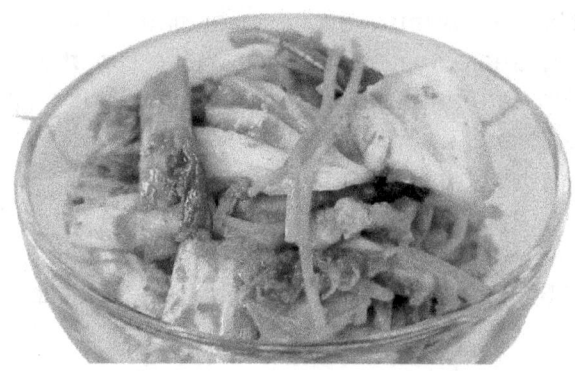

This bacteria naturally exists in the human digestive tract, but it can cause a pathogenic infection, which is one of the side effects of oral antibiotics. I also advised him that he could return to the doctor for additional medicines or try my natural healing method. He had no desire to obtain another antibiotic.

I had previously treated many people with C. diff. with wonderful results, so I was eager to make him feel better as soon as possible. I had him eliminate any inflammatory foods that were hurting his gut and feeding the C. diff bacteria as the first step. This is the anti-inflammatory diet I advocate in Chapter 3 of this book. I also advised him to use a natural herbal combination to treat his C. diff infection without aggravating his already inflamed intestines.

Second, we needed to re-inoculate his digestive system with lactic acid bacteria in order to quickly manage the C. diff. infection. He had tried probiotics in the past, but they had no effect. I emphasised that he needs far higher doses than what's generally seen in pills, and The Kimchi DietTM is the greatest method to receive high levels of probiotics. He was hesitant to prepare his own kimchi, but I assured him that if he followed my kimchi recipe and ate it as suggested, he would feel better. All he wanted was to have normal bowel movements back!

I saw him exactly ten days later, and I could tell by his expression that he was overjoyed to see me. After five days of consuming kimchi, his watery diarrhoea had ceased. The consistency was more like to "mud," and his bowel motions were reduced to three times per day. Furthermore, the sinus issues disappeared totally without the use of any medicine. Given everything he had been through for months, this was a significant step forward for him.

We stayed on The Kimchi DietTM for another two months, and not only did his C. diff. illness clear up entirely (as proven by another stool test) during the second month, but he also believes that kimchi saved his life. He still eats kimchi on a daily basis!

Inflammation is reduced.

Inflammation is one of the underlying causes of many of our ailments. As I explain in The 7-Day Allergy Makeover, when our body comes into contact with things that it can't simply handle, it frequently causes an inflammatory response. It's your body's way of fighting against these chemicals or toxins, much like when you're sick. If you consume enough processed foods or foods that you are sensitive to (gluten, dairy, sugar, soy, etc.), and live in an environment with dust mites, pet dander, or environmental pollutants, the inflammatory reaction might cause you to feel unwell and lethargic. It depletes your body's crucial resources for fighting real ailments when they do occur. It's why I've seen so many folks with allergies get sick every couple of months--their systems are expending all of their energy fighting allergies when they could be fighting disease. Not only that, but Kim et al. (2014) discovered a link between kimchi consumption and asthma incidence. Essentially, the more kimchi you consume, the lower your risk of developing asthma.[25] According to a 2016 study, rhinitis is the same.[26] For those who suffer from allergies, Rho et al. (2017) discovered that a specific bacterium found in kimchi called Enterococcus faecium FC-K has anti-allergenic benefits by lowering levels of IgE (Immunoglobulin E) in the body.[27] IgE is an essential marker for inflammation and allergies, therefore lower levels are beneficial.

Inflammation can also cause joint and muscular pain, edoema, and a variety of other discomforts. Chronic inflammation has been linked to arthritis, several autoimmune illnesses, and even some cancers. That's why, in Chapter 3, you'll learn about my Anti-Inflammatory Diet, a variant of what I offer to all of my patients because it nourishes your body with just the healthiest foods while eliminating as many potential irritants and allergies as possible. It's also the diet I used to heal my son Cody's allergies, and it's healed thousands of my patients suffering from allergies, arthritis, fibromyalgia, and autoimmune illnesses.

Of course, kimchi is an important part of my Anti-Inflammatory Diet. And the science backs it up. Not only does kimchi contain garlic and ginger, two of the strongest anti-inflammatory foods available, but cabbage in particular is a lesser-known anti-inflammatory and antioxidant meal. Kimchi also contains anti-inflammatory compounds that assist to protect the body from oxidative stress (which causes ageing and many diseases).[28] However, due to its probiotic component, kimchi has been demonstrated to aid with inflammation. Increasing probiotic intake is one of the most promising new areas of scientific research for managing inflammation, according to studies.[30] All of this suggests that replenishing your healthy gut flora with kimchi may be one of the most beneficial things you can do for your inflammation.

Autoimmune or Just Inflamed?

Sophia was a 36-year-old mother of 6-year-old twin boys and complained of sleep deprivation, constipation and muscle aches all over her body. She thought her stiffness and pain was from lack of exercise and the extra fifteen pounds of weight she'd not been able to shed since her pregnancy. She stated that she had a poor diet of sugar and snacks and didn't move around much– except when she was chasing after her boys!
Her physical exam was unremarkable except that her abdomen was bloated around her waistline. When I measured her waist and hip circumference, it was 36 inches in the waist and 34 inches in the hips. This indicated that her abdomen was either distended from an inflamed gut or from excess fat accumulation. Either way, she was not happy with her body and wanted to feel better.

I ordered all appropriate blood tests to rule out any issues including thyroid disease, anemia, blood sugar imbalances, autoimmune issues and more.

The only biomarker that was positive was the ANA, antinuclear antibodies test, which indicated that she was experiencing some form of autoimmune attack on her own tissues, hence the pain all over her body. I followed up with another blood test to find out what specific type of autoimmune disease it might point toward: rheumatoid arthritis, lupus, Sjogren's disease and so on. But all tests were negative, which was actually a good thing.

I suspected that she had gut issues and suffered from systemic inflammation from the poor eating habits. Lifestyle changes were in order.

I put her on The Kimchi Diet™, with some digestive supplements, and three weeks into our treatment protocol, Sophia's muscle pains had reduced by 75% and her constipation was completely gone. She confessed that she hadn't been this regular since she was in college! She also mentioned that she urinated excessively during the first two weeks, and that she lost a total of seven pounds in that short time. Unbelievable!

After eight weeks of The Kimchi Diet™, she came back into the office and wanted another blood test. Sophia was anxious to see if the ANA had changed, since she had been completely free of pain for weeks and was sleeping like a baby. Not only that, her belly was flatter and she had healthy bowel movements daily like clockwork. She had a lot more energy, was happier and ready to start a workout program at the local gym. I wasn't sure if the blood test would change so quickly, but I was pleasantly surprised that she passed her ANA blood test with flying colors!

Antioxidant Properties and Anti-Aging

As discussed, antioxidants are powerful compounds that help your body to fight oxidation or "rust" in the body by capturing free radicals. Free radicals are oxygen-containing molecules that bond easily with other chemicals in the body, setting off harmful chemical reactions and causing cellular damage. Just imagine your body trying going about its normal, healthy functions while it's bombarded with chemicals that can disrupt that functioning and cause degeneration. Now, keep in mind that even eating and breathing naturally cause some cellular damage over time, but we greatly speed this process up if we eat bad foods or are exposed to harmful toxicants and pollutants. Aging, at a simple level, is exactly this process of cellular damage caused by free radicals. Some have even suspected that if we could halt the work of free radicals in the body, we'd greatly slow the process of aging. It's why a fifty-year-old can be "younger" than a thirtyfive-year-old at the biological level: the healthy fifty-year-old has done less damage to their body in the form of free radical exposure and/or has consumed more foods with antioxidant properties. Free radical exposure comes in the form of:

- Pollution: Air and Water

- Heavy Metals and Chemicals

- Mold Toxicity

- Over the Counter and Prescription Drugs

- Smoking

- Alcohol

- Many Processed Meats

- Rancid Oils (Olive, Walnut, Avocado, Sesame and Coconut are the best)

- Lifestyle: Not Sleeping Enough, Exercising Too Much

Therefore, to reverse free radical impact and slow the process of aging, we need to minimize our exposure to the above compounds and foods, and we should include antioxidant foods like broccoli, cherries, spinach, blueberries and walnuts in our diet. And by now, you probably won't be surprised to learn that kimchi is one of the best antioxidative foods all around. Park and Ju (2018) show that kimchi has "vitamin C, chlorophyll, phenols, carotenoids, dietary fiber and other phytochemicals", as well as "further metabolites with

LAB (lactic acid bacteria)" that have antioxidant and anti-aging properties.[31] This anti-aging quality of kimchi increases as it ripens. Part of Korean folk wisdom is that eating well helps keep you feeling young–and now science has proven it! A new study suggests that kimchi consumption increases compounds like glutathione, the master antioxidant, which is anti-inflammatory and therefore may be helpful in treating and

Alzheimer's disease prevention (Woo et al. 2018).[32] It's also been demonstrated to be "neuroprotective" in mouse trials, aiding in nervous system regeneration.[33] Kimchi's high fibre content also contributes to its anti-aging properties. A high fibre diet has been linked to increased butyrate synthesis, a short-chain fatty acid (SCFA) produced by bacterial fermentation of fibre in the colon. Kimchi fibre feeds the lactic acid bacteria, and the metabolic end product increases butyrate. Butyrate is a short-chain fatty acid that has been linked to a reduction in colon disease such as cancer, brain inflammation, and other conditions. And butyrate has been associated to lower levels of inflammatory markers in the body.[34] This is critical for preventing ageing indications as we become older. Not only are the benefits of a high-fiber diet well-established for the colon, but there is now evidence that a high-fiber diet can positively impact gene expression in the brain, with the potential to treat many neurological illnesses that plague us as we age.[35] You've heard how vital fibre is your entire life, and here is your chance to consume plenty of it. Everyone gets a kimchi helping!

Better Digestion and Elimination

I am a firm believer that a healthy mind and body begin with proper digestion, but the majority of us lack this critical function. A weak digestive system can be caused by a variety of causes, including antibiotic use, excessive stress, a lack of quality sleep, and a diet high in processed foods. All sickness, they say, begins in the colon.

When we engage in these types of hazardous activities on a regular basis, our gut microbiome can become severely imbalanced, with too few "good guys" (probiotic bacteria) and too many "bad guys" (pathogenic bacteria, fungus, viruses, and parasites). When this happens, we can develop a wide range of symptoms, from constipation to bloating and gas to irritable bowel syndrome and chronic fatigue syndrome, as well as autoimmune illnesses and fibromyalgia. The possibilities are nearly limitless. As a result, millions of individuals suffer needlessly, frequently for many years.

Often, doctors will merely prescribe medications to treat the symptoms of these conditions, but these fast fixes rarely never address the underlying issue, which could be gut dysfunction. In addition to making healthy lifestyle choices like getting adequate sleep and properly managing stress, eating a diet rich in fresh and fermented whole foods can be extremely beneficial in conquering gut dysfunction and the diseases that often accompany it.

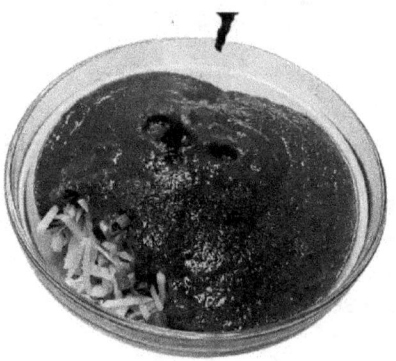

Kimchi is an excellent digestive aid, aiding in the breakdown of carbs and fibre in the grains and vegetables with which it is frequently consumed. The red pepper powder in kimchi stimulates stomach acid production, allowing us to digest our food more effectively. The lactic acid bacteria in kimchi aids in the breakdown of food and the equilibrium of our entire gut flora.[36] It has been demonstrated to lower the pH of the colon, which aids in the killing of dangerous organisms and reduces the amount of toxic enzymes.[37] As if that wasn't enough, Marco et al. (2017) discovered that bacteria found in fermented meals serve to protect against colitis and epithelial cell damage.[38] We currently only know about a fraction of the benefits that these small organisms provide to people, but we're learning more all the time.

Beware of Salmonellosis!

I'd been seeing Mark and his family for the past seven years, and they'd come in for everything from headaches to allergies to ordinary virus infections. However, I was asked if I could see Mark for an emergency visit this time. He had a business dinner at a sushi restaurant the night before and awoke in the middle of the night with terrible abdominal discomfort, cramping, and diarrhoea. He had gone to the toilet at least seven times before they phoned me early that morning because the diarrhoea wouldn't stop.

Even though this was most certainly a severe case of food poisoning, I wanted to send out a stool analysis. Stool tests, on the other hand, take time to get results, and I wanted to assist him as soon as possible. Mark was becoming weaker and experiencing headaches and chills with each round of diarrhoea.

Salmonella food poisoning is typically a self-limiting disease in which the patient is advised to rest, drink plenty of fluids, and eat a bland diet. If there is no bloody diarrhoea or a fever greater than 101.5 degrees Fahrenheit, the patient is sent home to care for themselves.

For a few days, I suggested Mark take oregano oil tablets, a natural antibacterial agent. I also requested Mark's wife, Kerry, to go to the grocery shop and get the napa cabbage kimchi with the most juice in the container. I had her squeeze out the kimchi juice from the cabbage and feed it to Mark every two hours until it was gone. I told them that he might have one more attack of diarrhoea, but that it would most likely stop after that. His cramping and gastrointestinal ache would be relieved by the kimchi juice.

Mark thanked me the next day, saying he had followed my advice exactly as advised. Sure enough, the kimchi juice worked! He did, in fact, experience one more round of diarrhoea, but it seemed more like a "purge." His stomach felt so comfortable and pleased that he went to bed early and woke up full of energy- fully cramp-free and diarrhea-free.

Kimchi to the rescue once more!

Diabetes, Heart Health, and Weight Loss

Almost everyone appears to be attempting to lose weight right now, often with little success. As of 2014, about one-third of the global population was overweight or obese, and if present trends continue, that figure will grow to nearly 50% by 2030.[39] We are all aware that being overweight or obese is a big contributor to a variety of health issues, including potentially fatal diseases such as cancer, heart disease, stroke, and diabetes. Obesity-related medical expenses in the United States alone were about $150 billion in 2014![40] And that's only for a year. What an unnecessary financial burden is being imposed on us. I bet that prices have only risen since 2014 and will continue to rise until we are able to control this epidemic.

The growth of processed foods over the previous century has had a significant role in the obesity epidemic in the United States. This comes as no surprise. In terms of encouraging health and energy, a diet rich in unprocessed, whole foods is the way to go. However, many people are unaware that fermented foods, which our forefathers consumed on a regular basis, are virtually entirely absent from most people's diets in this nation. And I feel that this is another major contributor to not only the number of people who are overweight or obese, but also to many other health conditions.

Numerous research in animals and people show that eating kimchi on a regular basis helps combat fat and overweight.[41] When you think about it, it makes logic. Kimchi is high in fibre, water, vitamins, minerals, phytochemicals, living enzymes, and good bacteria, yet low in fat and calories. Ideal diet food? Sure thing! When consumed on a daily basis, both fresh and fermented kimchi can reduce body weight, BMI, and body fat, although the effects of fermented kimchi are significantly stronger.[42] Furthermore, the red pepper powder used in many kimchi recipes contains capsaicin, a phytochemical that boosts our body's fat-burning metabolism. Garlic, radish, and ginger all play a role in weight loss, perhaps even more so than red pepper, thus even kimchi produced without red pepper can help people lose weight.[43] Good news for those of you who dislike spicy meals! Suffice it to say, kimchi is a nutritional powerhouse that should be on everyone's plate.

It was recently discovered that obese persons have a very different bacterial make-up in their digestive system than skinny people. However, kimchi has a good impact on the composition of our gut bacteria, particularly in obese people.[44] Scientists discovered that people who are overweight or obese have lower levels of Bacteroides and higher amounts of

Firmicutes, however eight weeks of regular kimchi eating was demonstrated to change this ratio favourably.[45] When an overweight person loses weight, the types and numbers of bacteria found in their gut alter dramatically, and vice versa when a thin person gains weight.[46] But here's the kicker: they discovered that consuming kimchi on a daily basis helps to modify the gut flora to match that of a skinny individual. Jackpot!

Along those lines, many fat people have diabetes, another condition caused by our contemporary lifestyle and its bad impact on our gut microbes. Diabetes affects an estimated 180 million individuals worldwide, although many of them are unaware that they have the disease.[47] Sugar (also found in refined carbs such as bread, pastries, spaghetti, and bagels) not only raises our blood sugar levels, but it also feeds the nasty bacteria in our stomach, as previously described. To feel normal, the body need an increasing amount of sugar. This may feel like brain fog or sugar crashes in less severe prediabetic situations. However, in more severe cases, the body becomes unable to regulate insulin production. Diabetes is the outcome. The good news is that kimchi--at least those made with napa cabbage--has been shown to help prevent diabetes in people who eat a high-fat diet.[48] Fresh and fermented kimchi can also help prediabetics lose weight, BMI (body mass index), waist circumference, insulin resistance, and blood pressure.[49] Heart health is a major concern for everyone who is overweight. Kimchi is also beneficial to overall heart health, as it lowers cholesterol and inflammation. One of kimchi's best qualities for a world plagued by obesity is its capacity to decrease cholesterol levels. A 2018 study discovered that some probiotic bacteria strains identified in kimchi decreased cholesterol in hypercholesterolemic rats. The microorganisms absorbed extra cholesterol while also causing the rats to expel it in their faeces.[50] In other words, they could handle some of the excess cholesterol while also disposing of some of it in their waste products. HDMPPA, an active component of kimchi, has also showed potential in reducing the development of fatty streaks in the aortic sinuses of rats fed a high cholesterol diet.[51] Another study found that, in addition to lowering cholesterol, kimchi lowers triglycerides and LDL levels, lessening the risk of a heart attack or stroke.[52] Kimchi can save our lives by reducing the amount of toxic substances in our systems. Kimchi has anti-atherosclerotic (heart protecting) characteristics and benefits in the body because it decreases cholesterol levels.[53] Kimchi promotes heart health!

It fascinates me to think of the trillions of gut bacteria that we all have in our bodies and to wonder what they're doing and why. Time will tell, but we've already begun to identify some of their key functions, and we know for certain that a healthy microbiome is a critical component of our general health and vitality. Millions of people fight year after year to reduce and keep off excess weight, and far too many of them fail despite their best efforts. Could kimchi and other fermented foods provide the missing link to long-term weight management? It is, without a doubt, a crucial component of a whole lifestyle transition that should not be overlooked.

Mood, Energy, and Mental Clarity

Consider how much you could accomplish if you had unlimited energy every day. Or if you could get through it all with a better attitude and mental clarity.

I normally go through my days with boundless energy, but this is because I've invested so much time and energy in my health over the years. However, plentiful energy was not always the norm for me, and it is certainly not the usual for the majority of the individuals who come to me for health advice. We're all overworked and overstressed, and it's costing us dearly.

However, aside from job and stress (all of which have an impact on how much energy you have), what you eat has a significant impact on how much energy you have throughout the day. Ideally, you should consume several meals and snacks each day that include unprocessed foods such as fresh fruits and vegetables, nuts and seeds, gluten-free whole grains, and clean protein, as well as a healthy dosage of fermented foods such as kimchi. All of this is covered in Chapter 3 of my Anti-Inflammatory Diet, and I go into greater detail in The 7-Day Allergy Makeover. A combination of these meals will give your body with a healthy balance of carbohydrates, protein, and fat, as well as the micronutrients it need to function efficiently over time.

More than 8% of adults in the United States are depressed, and women are twice as likely as men to be affected.[54] If you or someone you know has struggled with depression, you understand how difficult it can be. Anxiety disorders, on the other hand, are the most frequent mental ailment in the United States, affecting over 18% of the population each year. And the gut biome serves as a physiological link between what we eat and how we feel. The vagus nerve, which goes from the gut to the brain, connects our mind to our internal flora, delivering messages back and forth. More research indicates that the "gastrointestinal tract is emotionally sensitive." Anger, worry, grief, and elation are all emotions that can cause discomfort in the gut."[55] As a result, anxiety can create gut reactions, but gut disorders can also cause anxiety or depression. This helps to explain why, according to John Hopkins University, a higher percentage of people with IBS develop anxiety or depression than a random sample of the population.[56]

There's good news, however. Dinan et. al (2013) have come to define a new category of food, psychobiotics, which consists of a "live organism that, when ingested in adequate amounts, produces a health benefit in patients suffering from psychiatric illness. These bacteria, as a kind of probiotic, are capable of generating and distributing neuroactive chemicals including gamma-aminobutyric acid (GABA) and serotonin, which operate on the brain-gut axis."[57] Since a large variety of antidepressants already work to increase serotonin production (or inhibit its reuptake), Dinan's research opens–or verifies–the connection Koreans have understood between eating kimchi and improved emotional state. But the connection between kimchi and mood goes even further. Specific bacteria present in kimchi have been found to increase GABA production in our brains, also verifying Dinan's research.[58] GABA is a neurotransmitter that's known to induce calmness and relaxation and helps to relieve depression, anxiety, insomnia and more. Lactic acid bacteria isolated from kimchi increase the production of gamma-aminobutyric acid (GABA), which also has a neuroprotective effect on the brain.[59] Getting your gut right with healthy bacteria that come from kimchi will do a lot to enhance your mood and give you that feeling of relaxation and release from pressure we Koreans call siwonhan-mat.

Clear Skin

Who wouldn't want clearer and more radiant skin? By making kimchi a regular part of your diet, your skin will receive a huge boost of nutrients to help it detoxify wastes, retain moisture and maintain an even skin tone. As discussed above, kimchi kicks inflammation to the curb like yesterday's trash. And inflammation is your skin's worst enemy, so anything that cools and soothes your skin from the inside out is worth its weight in gold!

High kimchi consumption (eaten at most meals) has been linked to lower incidence of eczema (atopic dermatitis), while high consumption of processed foods and meat has been linked to a higher incidence of eczema, a skin disorder that's always puzzled the medical community as to its cause and how to heal it.[60] In animal studies, kimchi was shown to directly help promote healthy skin conditions.[61] In particular, one study found that 3-5 oz. (2-4 servings) of kimchi per day significantly reduced the incidence of atopic dermatitis in adults.[62] Kimchi does this by significantly altering our gut bacteria,[63] and using lactic acid bacteria topically can also improve this skin condition.[64] Finally, since acne is all about inflammation, we want to do everything we can to lower it by addressing the gut. Between the diet program I recommend in the next chapter and an increase in probiotics, kimchi works to heal dysbiosis and the intestinal issues that cause inflammation. Plus, with its anti-inflammatory ingredients like ginger and garlic, you'll be set for beautiful, radiant skin!

Acne or Mites?

Daniel was a lovely 17-year-old teenager and had been battling cystic acne since she was twelve. The acne covered her forehead, cheeks and chest. Her mother

Daphne had already taken her to five different dermatologists before coming to my office. Daniel had tried their topical medications and skin care products, only to find that some worked for a little while and some made things worse. The doctors all told her mother that Daniel needed to be on oral antibiotics, but she was reluctant to put her daughter on them because Daniel had an allergic reaction to penicillin as a child. They came to see me because Daniel was desperate to have clear skin.

When I looked closer with a high-powered magnification loupes (surgical glasses), I noticed that some areas on her face looked like true acne, but other areas did not. Many areas were red and inflamed but without pustules. I suspected she actually had demodex mites in her skin, and this didn't sit well with Daniel or her mother. I wanted her to get it checked out under a microscope with her dermatologist, but they declined.

I mentioned that Daniel's skin microbiome was completely out of balance. The pH of her skin was too acidic, causing acne breakouts. There was also the secondary issue of microscopic demodex mites living in her follicle and oil glands, causing more inflammation and irritation. We had to change her skin microbiome quickly, and to do that, I recommended we heal her gut first with The Kimchi Diet™. Skin problems often stem from an unhealthy gut.

When I mentioned to Daniel that she'd have to start on The Kimchi Diet™, she was actually very happy with the treatment protocol. Her best friend Sunny was Korean and Daniel loved going over for home-cooked meals and kimchi. My goal was to shift her internal and external skin microbiome, so that her immunity would be stronger and healthier from the inside out. I also changed her daily skin care routine and recommended that she needed to sweat more to open up her pores through exercise and steam facials.

Within two weeks on The Kimchi Diet™ and the all-natural Purigenex® skin care regimen, Daniel came back into the office with a huge smile on her face and gave me the biggest hug! The large cystic acne spots were healing and the discolorations and irritations were returning back to healthier-looking skin. There weren't any new acne spots either. Emotionally, she was feeling better about herself. Acne flare-ups triggered by her hormonal fluctuations (especially around her menstrual cycle) still affected her, so it took a total of three months to completely clear up.

Daniel still eats kimchi daily and her acne scars are long gone, replaced by the beautiful vibrant skin she always dreamed of.

Cancer Treatment and Prevention

While cancer prevention requires a comprehensive lifestyle of minimising exposure to carcinogens, there are functional foods we can eat to help our bodies avoid its growth. To prevent cancer, it is critical to avoid smoking and drinking, as well as contact with hazardous chemicals and pesticides. Kimchi, on the other hand, can have a role in cancer prevention through a healthy lifestyle shift. According to Park and Ju (2018), "administration of kimchi may be helpful for lowering faecal pH and deactivation of hazardous enteric enzymes, which may result in maintaining good colon health and suppressing the formation of carcinogens, and eventually promote colon health and colorectal cancer prevention," and that even dead lactic acid bacteria from kimchi "prevented colitis and colon cancer in animal studies."[65] The usage of Chinese pepper and organic cabbage boosted this effect. Their findings also reveal that kimchi inhibits cancer cell proliferation while having no negative effects on normal cells. Kimchi has been found in additional studies to have anti-cancer effects on pancreatic and liver cancer cells, with a stronger effect on pancreatic cancer, which has historically been one of the more difficult to cure types of cancer.[66] However, the benefits of kimchi do not end there. Other researchers believe it can help with both cancer prevention and treatment.

[67] Kimchi is a wonder meal that should be included in a global health-food movement.

Blood Pressure Control

With all of the salt, you might think kimchi is terrible for your blood pressure. You are not alone. Many Koreans have recently begun to reduce their kimchi consumption in response to research linking excessive kimchi consumption to hypertension. However, a recent study found no definitive link between kimchi eating and hypertension.[68] The experts who conducted the study believe that the high potassium content of kimchi serves to balance out the sodium, resulting in no harmful effects on blood pressure. So, go ahead and eat your kimchi every day without worrying about your blood pressure, but check with your doctor first!

In fact, the numerous vitamins, minerals, enzymes, and phytochemicals included in kimchi will aid in the attainment and maintenance of healthy blood pressure.

Now that we've learned everything there is to know about the history of kimchi and its nearly limitless health advantages, the only thing left to do is start preparing and eating kimchi on a daily basis. It couldn't be a more basic lifestyle modification to implement, but it can have life-changing consequences for you and your family.

Chapter 3: Kimchi Diet

Preparation Phase: A Commitment to Healthful Eating

As you begin The Kimchi Diet™, it's important to eat as healthily as possible. Just think about it: kimchi may be a very powerful superfood, but no superfood alone can possibly have its full effects if your body is having to spend its energy processing bad food. Unfortunately, the standard American diet is chock-full of foods that are difficult for the body to deal with. From processed foods to refined sugars to deep fried foods, sometimes it seems our whole diet is meant to put a stress on the system. These foods may not produce a noticeable effect if you only eat them once a year. But if you eat them every week, they can produce inflammatory responses–as if your body thinks it's sick! Even though you may not have a full-blown anaphylactic or IgE reaction, the body slowly becomes inflamed and spends its valuable resources trying to "fight" these food stressors, instead of spending all its vital energy on mental function, hormone regulation, pumping blood, and so forth.

In the course of thirty years, working with patients suffering from allergies, irritable bowel syndrome, chronic fatigue and more, I've developed an Anti-Inflammatory Nutrition Plan that's meant to help reduce inflammation quickly and make the body feel vibrant, so it can run at its optimal capacity. It's the one I detail in The 7-Day Allergy Makeover, the one that helped my son, Cody to overcome his lifethreatening allergies, and the same one (with some key additions) that I used to help my recovery from brain injury, as I talk about in The Mighty Mito. This is not a crash diet, cleanse, detox or quick fix. It's a nutrition plan to follow for the rest of your life, because it embodies the best of healthy eating from my clinical experience and research over the years. So even if you haven't read those books, I want to give you the condensed version of my Anti-Inflammatory Nutrition Plan here.

The Anti-Inflammatory Nutrition Plan

To begin with, the simple rule to follow is this: eat whole, natural, unprocessed and organic foods. Vegetables, fruits, free-range meat, nuts, seeds and ancient grains like quinoa and amaranth are all great options. In general, try to fill half your plate with veggies (this is where the kimchi comes in!), a quarter of it with protein (beans, meat) and a quarter of it with healthful grains. Top it off with good fats like olive oil or avocado. Just following this one simple rule can change so much for so many Americans!

Beyond that, there are four food groups that I recommend eliminating completely from your diet: gluten products, dairy, sugars (including alcohol) and artificial, highly processed ingredients. In my clinical practice and medical research, I've found that many people are extremely sensitive to these foods, often without knowing it. These foods often cause hidden inflammatory reactions in the gut–leading to inflammation and increased permeability in the gut lining, known as "leaky gut syndrome." Furthermore, everything from brain fog, energy crashes and rashes all the way up to acid reflux, bloating, diarrhea and vomiting have been traced back to the consumption of certain foods in this group among some of my patients. Let me briefly detail what to cut out and most importantly, why.

Gluten Products

Gluten is what makes bread and wheat "chewy" and is especially difficult for our digestive system to process, due to the high levels of fructans–long chains of fructose molecules. Not to mention that most commercially produced wheat is sprayed with an herbicide made of glyphosate, possibly the worst herbicide out there. Therefore, please eliminate:

- Wheat (whole and white)

- Oats (unless specified as gluten-free)

- Barley

- Pasta

- Spelt

  Kamut

- Bread and bagels

- Donuts

- Rye

Nowadays, you can find many gluten-free foods, from pizza crusts to pasta to bread. Make sure that these are made of quinoa, brown rice, wild rice, corn or amaranth. Still it's best to limit your consumption of these foods, as they can also lead to inflammation. You might try replacing them with a vegetable like cauliflower, which can often work well with recipes that call for grains.

Dairy Products

Along with the gluten-free revolution, the dairy-free revolution has hit the United States hard in the last decade. The majority of the population after the age of five is lactose intolerant due to the lack of lactase enzyme production by the brush borders of the small intestine. Without the ability to digest lactose, people's bodies are irritated by the undigested sugar in milk. It can cause an overgrowth of bacteria and yeast, triggering irritable bowel symptoms such as gas, bloating, cramping and diarrhea. As mentioned above, leaky gut syndrome is caused by the inflammatory response of too much sugar. Dairy can contribute to this syndrome as well.

Traditional Korean cuisine is both gluten-free and dairy-free. If you go to a Korean restaurant, you will see some foods made with wheat or milk, but these are due to the more recent history of Westernization. 99% of Korean food is still based on gluten-free and dairy-free recipes.

Eliminating dairy products means cutting out anything made with cow's, sheep's or goat's milk.

- Milk

- Cheese

- Ice Cream

- Yogurt

- Sour Cream

- Cream Cheese

- Dairy Salad Dressings or Sauces

Instead, try the many unsweetened alternatives made from rice, almond, walnut (my favorite), hazelnut, coconut or hemp. Some people are reactive to soy products, so I can't recommend soy milk for everyone. Many people mistake eggs for a dairy product, but they should not be put in this category. Eggs are a great source of protein–although once again–many of my patients have been sensitive to them. If you're not, I certainly encourage you to eat eggs from pasture-raised organic chickens.

Sugars

With all the problems that we face from diabetes and Alzheimer's, it's no wonder that sugar is at the top of many doctors' "Do Not Eat" list. But as the market gets flooded with supposedly more healthful alternatives, many people are confused about what's okay and what's not okay to consume.

Here's my simple formula: do your best to not eat any sweetener, even if it's all natural, like honey or agave. Sugar and refined carbs (like white rice) spike the blood sugar and lead to energy crashes and brain fog, or if consumed in high enough quantities, insulin resistance. That's right, foods like white pasta or white bread are almost entirely simple sugars at the end of the day, so I recommend eliminating them. Cutting out sugar is one of the single best things you can do for your health.

Now, with that said, you'll notice that sugar can be one of the ingredients in kimchi recipes. So why is that? The sugar is something added–usually one teaspoon–for the lactic acid bacteria to feed on. Once they feed on it, however, you are not actually ingesting the sugar, but rather the byproducts of the fermentation process itself. The point of this sugar is not to increase calories, but simply to allow the lactic acid bacteria to grow, and it does provide a slightly sweeter taste. Once again, the sugar in kimchi is completely optional.

- Sugar (White, Brown, Raw, Turbinado)

- Honey

- Molasses

- Evaporated Cane Juice

- Agave Nectar

- Coconut Sugar

- Date Sugar

- Maple Syrup

- White rice

- White bread and pasta (Contain Gluten) Alcohol

Some monk fruit and erythritol sweeteners are good options. Stevia is ok too. Just make sure they have nothing else added. Some even have lactose—which is a dairy product, so beware!

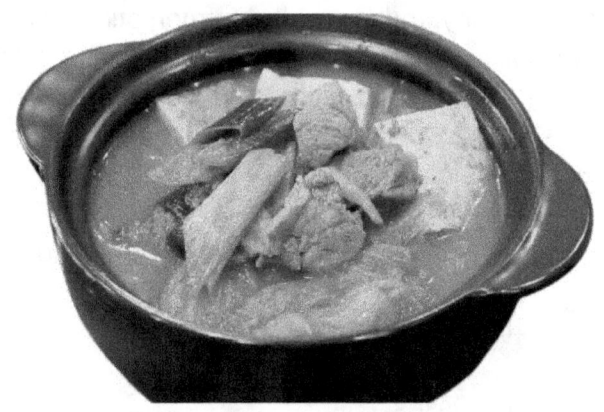

Food Additives and Highly Processed Ingredients

Finally, we get to food additives, which really aren't foods at all. These are chemicals used to make food look better, stay preserved longer, or supposedly taste better. Some, like high fructose corn syrup, come from natural sources but have no nutritional value. There's no reason to eat these, and considering what a toxic burden they add to the body, there's almost nothing you can do to improve your health more than refrain from eating the following:

- Aspartame (Nutrasweet®, blue packet)

- Sucralose (Splenda®, yellow packet)

- Saccharin (Sweet 'N Low®, pink packet)

- High Fructose Corn Syrup

- MSG (monosodium glutamate)

- Food Coloring (red, blue, yellow dyes)

- Nitrites (sausage, deli meats)

- Sulfites (wine, beer, deli food)

- BHA (pork sausages, chips, instant tea, packaged food)

- Butylates or BHT (butter, vegetable oils, margarine)

- Benzoates (fruit juices, ketchup, tea, coffee)

- Hydrogenated Oils (margarine, vegetable shortening, packaged snacks)

In addition to these foods, I recommend that people who are especially prone to allergies or have digestive issues consider cutting out eggs, peanuts, mushrooms and soy products. You can then try reintroducing them one by one to see if you have any reactions. If not, feel free to enjoy them in your daily life. For more information on the Anti-Inflammatory Nutrition Plan, check out The 7-Day Allergy Makeover or the Resource section.

Those with Irritable Bowel Syndrome or Gut Issues

If you've been diagnosed with irritable bowel syndrome or often experience bloating, gas, poor digestion or constipation, you should modify the above diet to help your gut bacteria "reset." Often, these symptoms are the result of an overload of what are known as fermentable carbohydrates—namely, foods that bacteria in the gut help our body to process. In addition, when you eat too many fermentable carbohydrates or don't have enough helpful gut bacteria, this process can become less efficient, resulting in an overload of gas—which is a byproduct of bacterial fermentation. So what's the way out of this conundrum?

I advocate the Anti-Inflammatory Nutrition Plan stated above, but with a twist. You should also limit your consumption of fermentable carbohydrates, generally known as FODMAP meals. This abbreviation stands for Fermentable Oligosaccharides, Disaccharides, Monosaccharides, and Polyols, which are the carbohydrates that our bodies ferment. Because the human body lacks the enzymes needed to break down these sugars, they must be fermented in the gut. Irritable bowel symptoms may arise if too many FODMAP foods are consumed, particularly if there is an excess of harmful bacteria or fungi. Reducing your intake of fermentable carbs at the start of The Kimchi DietTM will soothe your gut, boost your energy, and reduce other symptoms.

While the lists below are not thorough, they do give you an idea of which foods to avoid. I've merged the Anti-Inflammatory Nutrition Plan and the FODMAPFree Diet to create The Ultimate Wellness for Life Food List, which is available in the Resource section.

FODMAP Foods

The following are FODMAP foods that I have all of my patients exclude as part of the usual Anti-Inflammatory Nutrition Plan:

- Sugars

- Alcohol

- Gluten Grains

- Dairy Products

Furthermore, if you have IBS, you should avoid several healthy meals that are high in fermentable carbohydrates:

- Beans

- Soy Products

- Cabbage

- Cruciferous Vegetables (Broccoli, Cauliflower)

- Artichokes

- Asparagus

- Apples

- Cherries

- Pears

- Watermelon

- Apricots

- Prunes

These are all generally healthful foods (with the possible exception of soy for some people). However, if you have a bacterial overgrowth, the excess bacteria will feed on these meals, causing gas and bloating because the body lacks the enzymes needed to break them down.

Remove them from your diet for four to six weeks to reduce bacterial overgrowth, depending on when you start feeling better. Then, one by one, gradually reintroduce them into your diet. Keep in mind that fermentable carbs cannot be completely eliminated. If you have a bacterial overgrowth and irritable bowel symptoms, you should only use them for a short period of time. Consider this a component of your gut healing programme.

To accommodate everyone, I purposefully created The Kimchi DietTM to begin with lower-FODMAP foods (like cucumbers) and end with higher-FODMAP foods (like cabbage). Even those with healthy guts can become overwhelmed if they start eating cabbage every day! The good news is that there is virtually nothing better you can do to help your irritable bowel symptoms than consume kimchi, since its beneficial microorganisms will work to digest FODMAP foods.

Although I'm asking you to eliminate inflammatory foods from your diet for faster results, I'd like to emphasise that The Kimchi DietTM is about incorporating kimchi into whatever diet you're on, whether it's meat and potatoes or a vegan diet.

This is not about deprivation, but rather about health through addition.

If eliminating all of these inflammatory items is too tough for you or your family, then eliminate just one of the following groups: gluten grains, sweets, or dairy foods. When you start experiencing great results, it may be simpler to get rid of the next food offender and feel more inspired to make meaningful lifelong changes. While the perfect nutrition programme may be sugar-free, gluten-free, dairy-free, organic, and free of food additives, it may take your family some time to get there--and that's fine. True health is a long-term process!

The 8-Week Kimchi Diet

Our eight-week journey into the amazing world of kimchi begins here. What follows is a strategy I've developed over the years for introducing my patients to this miracle food while minimising stomach upset and ensuring a continual supply of new kimchi tastes and flavours. It has helped to lessen allergies, clear up acne, produce weight reduction, reduce pain and inflammation, and enhance energy and mental clarity.

Furthermore, The Kimchi DietTM's magic lies in the ideal levels of lactic acid bacteria you'll be consuming on a regular basis. You can always experiment with new vegetables or kimchi variations. But by starting with this 8-week regimen, you'll have a wonderful head start on improving your gut biome and your health with the power of kimchi.

Although I've provided you with a chronological schedule for The Kimchi DietTM 8-week plan, don't feel obligated to follow it precisely as it's put out. Some of my patients require extra time to heal their gut and may require sixteen weeks instead of eight--no issue! Move at your own pace, as you know best how quickly you can transition from one phase to the next. Actually, your instincts will tell you!

To maximise the health advantages of kimchi, the most important schedule to follow is consuming the proper sort of kimchi from the outset, and in a sequential way from Phase 1 to Phase 4. The amount of time between each phase isn't as vital as eating kimchi every day for gut healing success!

As I detail each phase of The Kimchi DietTM below, I encourage that you also read The Kimchi DietTM Recipe chapter to become acquainted with each variety of kimchi, as there are a lot of instructive photographs that will be very helpful. Visuals make things so much easier to understand!

Timeline of The Kimchi Diet in Brief

Days 1-14 of Phase 1

Make Cucumber Kimchi on Day 1.

Day 3-4: Begin eating 2–3 pieces of one cucumber kimchi floret per day.

Day 7-8: Work your way up to eating a full cucumber kimchi floret every day.

Day 8: Make kimchi with baby bok choy, mustard greens, radish tops or beetroot tops.

Day 8-14: Continue to consume 1 cucumber kimchi floret per day.

Phase 2: 14-28 days

Day 14-21: Finish the cucumber kimchi and begin eating 1 tablespoon of your preferred Phase 2 kimchi (baby bok choy, mustard greens, radish tops or beetroot tops), gradually increasing to two teaspoons per day.

Make root vegetable kimchi (radish, daikon, turnip or rutabaga kimchi) on day 21.

Day 21-28: Eat Phase 2 kimchi as usual.

Phase 3: 28-42 days

Day 28: Continue to eat one to two teaspoons of the root vegetable kimchi (radish, daikon, turnip or rutabaga kimchi) and finish the Phase 2 kimchi.

Make the napa cabbage kimchi on Day 28.

Day 28-42: Eat 2-3 tablespoons of both Phase 2 and Phase 3 kimchi per day.

Days 42-56 and Beyond in Phase 4

Day 42: Consume one to two teaspoons of napa cabbage kimchi while keeping an eye out for symptoms.

Day 42-56: Continue eating the leftover Phase 2 and Phase 3 kimchi and introducing napa cabbage kimchi into your diet. Work your way up to 4 tablespoons of kimchi every day.

Four tablespoons equals a quarter cup of kimchi, which means you'll be consuming more than 60 billion CFUs of lactic acid bacteria per day!

Days 1-14 of Phase 1

Make sure you have all of the necessary Kimchi Tools on Day 1 (or earlier):

- Knife with a Sharp Edge

- chopping board

- Mixing Bowl, Large

- Colander

- Grater for Fruit

- Gloves and an apron (to protect your hands from the red pepper powder and kimchi paste)

- Mason jars or airtight containers made of glass

- Containers made of earthenware (optional if you prefer glass)

Then, go to the store and acquire the following kimchi ingredients: solar sea salt, garlic, ginger, coarse red pepper powder, Asian pears (Bosc pears are great), Fuji apples, and spring onions. This week, you'll make Cucumber Kimchi, a quick and easy kimchi that you can eat within a few days. Purchase some cucumbers as well. You can make it as mild or spicy as you like, but keep in mind that many of the good bacteria and health benefits of kimchi are derived from red pepper powder, so try to include it if feasible. Spicy kimchi is really delicious to me!

Although Cucumber Kimchi can be eaten right away, as many Koreans do, to maximise the health benefits of the LAB and phytonutrients, allow fermentation to take place first!

Take one floret from the bottom of the jar on Day 3 or 4 to guarantee you're getting the healthy bacteria in the juices.

Remove each cucumber leaf from the stem and cut it into bite-sized pieces. Eat no more than three to four pieces per day, as a side dish or salad with lunch or dinner.

At this point, a modest level of lactic acid bacteria has been formed, making it simple to incorporate Cucumber Kimchi into your diet.

Serve your roasted chicken with a piece of cucumber kimchi on top, add it to vegetables to enhance the flavour, or serve it over quinoa or inside a taco. It's even good with scrambled eggs!

During the first few days of fermentation, the kimchi will taste like seasoned raw cucumbers, but after a week, as the fermentation process progresses, you will be rewarded with a tangy, somewhat sweet, powerful, spicy flavour! That is the bacteria at work.

Enjoy the development of flavours as it progresses from mild to completely mature, and your kimchi taste buds will be refined in no time!

Beginning on Day 8, make Bok Choy, Beet Tops, Mustard Green Tops or Radish Tops Kimchi (whatever is most readily available in markets). Again, mild or spicy is acceptable. This kimchi will not be eaten straight away; instead, it will ferment for a week before being consumed. Then, on day fourteen, you can begin consuming them as the Cucumber Kimchi finishes.

As the Cucumber Kimchi ferments in the refrigerator for the next two weeks, the LAB population will steadily increase, eventually reaching up to 1 billion CFUs per gramme of kimchi.

By the end of Day 10 to 14, you should be able to eat one complete cucumber floret twice a day.

Cucumber Kimchi is best eaten within three weeks of making it since it loses its crunchy texture and can become extremely sour after that. It will not "go bad" if it is a month old, but the texture will become soft and mushy. Cucumber kimchi juice is still safe to consume; it's tasty and high in probiotics.

One tablespoon of kimchi every day will keep the doctor away!

By the way, if you can't consume spicy dishes, don't worry! Kimchi can be made without the red pepper. In fact, for the first 1700 years, kimchi was cooked without red pepper. At the end of each recipe in Chapter 5, I've included additional instructions on how to create the recipe without the red pepper powder. Without the red pepper, the fermentation process will go faster, and you may need to place it in the refrigerated sooner, perhaps 6 to 8 hours after the initial ambient temperature fermentation. You'll also need to consume the non-spicy kimchi you prepare faster than the hot ones.

Don't be concerned if you notice things churning in your intestines during Phase 1. You'll be relieved to know that there's a "bug war" going on in your gut during the first few weeks, but it's working in your favour. The LAB contained in kimchi naturally helps to eradicate bad bacteria in your digestive tract, and there will be a brief period of microbial hierarchy battle. But in the end, the good guys will be king. However, if you experience excessive bloating, gas, burping, abdominal cramping or diarrhoea after incorporating cucumber kimchi into your diet, I recommend you stop for a few days or until the symptoms have subsided, and then reintroduce it into your diet, but only half the amount daily, or every other day.

KIMCHI TIP: How to Get Rid of Kimchi Breath?

Some people perceive a little garlicky odour on their breath after eating kimchi. That one is also solved. My secret ingredient is ginger!

I discovered this kimchi breath remedy many years ago when researching one of my PurigenexTM skin care products, Age Reverse Serum. Liposomal glutathione, a great antioxidant and anti-aging cosmeceutical, was one crucial ingredient I wanted to include in the formula, but it had a strong sulphur flavour.

I must have tried over fifty different natural perfumes to disguise the sulphur smell before settling on ginger.

Since then, I've been drinking ginger tea directly after eating kimchi, which is pretty much after every meal. I even keep a tiny container of organic ginger powder in my purse in case we go to the neighbourhood Korean eatery. Not only will it freshen your breath, but it will also provide some of the fantastic health advantages of ginger, which is an antioxidant, anti-inflammatory, sugar balancer, and more!

Kimchi Breath Remedy

Dissolve 1/4 teaspoon ginger in 10 oz. of hot or cold water and drink after eating any type of kimchi. This ginger drink will also help with garlic and onion breath!

Phase 2: Days 14-28

By Day 14, you may have eaten most of the Cucumber Kimchi, and if it's extremely ripe--that is, if it tastes sour and has lost its crunchiness--you can compost or toss it. If it still tastes good, keep eating little amounts of it and gradually incorporate Mustard Greens or Radish Tops Kimchi into your diet.

After just one week of fermentation, your second batch of kimchi should be ready to eat on Day 14. Begin with one tablespoon every day, with lunch or dinner. As the days pass, if you feel good and your body and intestinal tract allow it (no allergic responses, bloating, gas or indigestion), consume a tablespoon of the kimchi twice each day--once with lunch and once with dinner.

Continue to consume up to two teaspoons of the Mustard Greens or Radish Tops Kimchi for the following two weeks (Days 14-28). The kimchi will be fully ripe, and the kimchi microbiota will be at its peak. At this time, sourness should be kept to a minimum.

Starting on Day 21, make a root vegetable kimchi with daikon, turnip, and carrot.

Rutabaga or radish Kimchi to be eaten a week later: Day 28 or so

(138). My favourite is Korean Radish, and my second favourite is Daikon (more narrow)--but experiment and discover your own! Most kimchi takes a week or two to prepare, with the exception of cucumber and other lighter veggies.

As previously said, continue eating two teaspoons of Mustard Greens, Beet Tops, Bok Choy or Radish Tops Kimchi each day, and if you feel your gut is ready, add one tablespoon of Root Vegetable Kimchi per day around Day 28. If you encounter any discomfort, you can always return to two tablespoons of Phase 1 or Phase 2 kimchi every day. The Kimchi DietTM is a customised regimen that you may follow at your own speed to meet your specific health needs.

Phase 3: 28-42 days

Radish Kimchi or another hard root vegetable will last you two to four weeks. From Day 28 to 42, eat two teaspoons with your lunch and dinner. These root veggies can be stored for four to six weeks, or even longer, depending on how much you create and consume. Radish Kimchi juice is traditionally used to treat diarrhoea and constipation. I keep two or three bottles of the leftover juice in my fridge and take a tablespoon here and there for the refreshing taste and the lactic acid bacteria.

You've probably been inoculating your digestive tract with billions of lactic bacteria every day by now. Remember that one gramme of kimchi contains approximately one billion CFUs (colony forming units) of beneficial bacteria, so you're on a roll.

Around this time, many people start to detect changes in their bodies. You may notice that your stomach feels lighter, less bloated, less worried, or that you have more energy. Don't worry if you don't. It may take some time to notice a difference, especially if your gut microbiota is reduced. Beginning on Day 28, prepare Napa Cabbage Kimchi for the sixth week of The Kimchi DietTM. This is the kimchi that most people envision when they think of kimchi, and it's also my personal favourite. Something about the crunchy cabbage, the heat, and the garlic and ginger always wins me over. This kimchi requires a little more time than the others, not because it takes longer to ferment, but because the extra time allows the LAB to predigest the napa cabbage for a longer period of time, lowering the fermentable carbohydrate levels. This will reduce gas and bloating problems.

Days 42-56 and Beyond in Phase 4

Napa Kimchi is the litmus test for determining the health of your gut microbiota. On Day 42, begin consuming it one tablespoon at a time. If your microbiome is still out of balance, you will experience a lot of gas, bloating, and frequent bowel movements, as well as loose stool. If this is the case, reduce the Napa Cabbage Kimchi and continue with the other kimchi. Simply re-create the Cucumber Kimchi for a quick snack, or return to Mustard Greens or Radishes--your pick.

If everything goes well, you should keep eating the Napa Kimchi--it's possibly the most potent variety for restoring the gut microbiota. Consume one to two tablespoons daily for the next two weeks, or until Day 56. Check in with yourself at that point. What are your feelings now compared to when you started? Do you have more energy, are you more attentive, and are you in a better mood? Have you lost weight or do you feel more at ease in your own skin? These are all indicators that The Kimchi DietTM is working!

If you feel particularly wonderful, consider gradually increasing to four tablespoons of kimchi per day, divided between two meals. Four tablespoons equals around a quarter cup of kimchi, so you'd be consuming more than 60 billion CFUs of various lactic acid bacteria per day.

However, The Kimchi DietTM does not finish after eight weeks! Including kimchi in your daily meals is one of the nicest things you can do for your family. I recommend keeping some Napa Cabbage or Radish Kimchi on hand at all times. Plus, if you run out of fresh vegetables for your next meal, kimchi is always accessible to help you meet your daily vegetable requirement!

I normally prepare a new batch of kimchi every two weeks and have a variety of bottles of kimchi in various states of fermentation in my kimchi refrigerator, including some that are three months old, yum!

That's part of the fun of kimchi: you can prepare it with whatever vegetables you like and have it ready to go in a week or two with no cooking and nearly no effort.

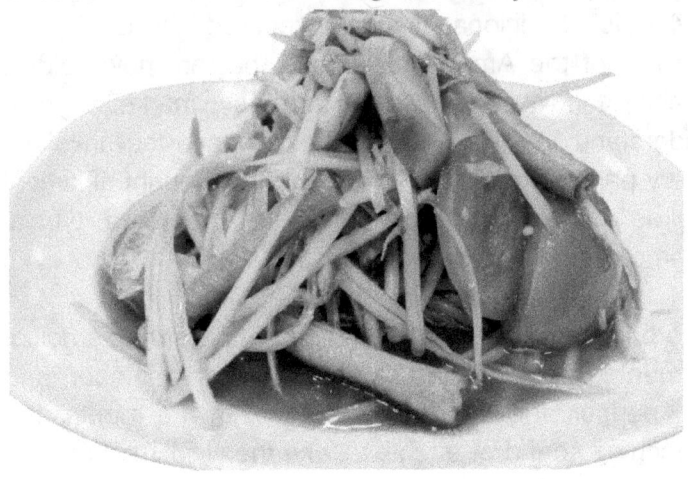

Chapter 4: An Overview on how to make Kimchi

The Kimchi Diet plan is now complete, so let's take a quick look at how to produce kimchi. Although the book's recipe section, Chapter 5, contains detailed instructions on how to produce different types of kimchi, this chapter includes some basic guidelines and advice for making kimchi.

If you've ever tasted kimchi—I'm talking about real, authentic, traditional kimchi prepared by a Korean family, not the American variants that are now sold in health food shops and farmers' markets—you'll understand that it's a sensory experience that involves every part of your body. Even now, the thought of kimchi makes my mouth start to water—this is a typical example of a Pavlovian response!

The bubbling sweet and sour flavour, the strong smell of fermented vegetables, the aroma of garlic, ginger, and red pepper, the cool and crisp feel in the mouth, the crunching sound of each bite, and the vivid Technicolour of red, white, and green of the vegetables all fully activate all of my senses as if I'm eating a big bite of it.

In the following two chapters, I hope to share with you the kimchi culture that has been handed down from mother to daughter over many generations, enabling you to not only reap the many health benefits of kimchi but also to eat it as my mother and her predecessors intended. I want you to feel the full-body sense of contentment that we Koreans refer to as siwonhan-mat, an untranslatable word that means "relief from pressure" or "physical calibration", specifically after enjoying a good meal. This feeling will be familiar to everyone who has eaten in a Korean restaurant or at the home of a Korean friend. I'm hoping that the kimchi recipes I learned from my grandma, mother, and myself would give you all of this and more.

Making Kimchi in Culture

It goes like this in an old Korean proverb: "The best kimchi flavour depends on oemoni's sohn, or "mother's hand." And in our large family, the tastiest kimchi was produced by Halmeoni's Sohn (grandmother's hand). Naturally, the elder received the honour because they are revered as the wise and respected members of all indigenous communities. I'm sure kimchi played a role in the 104 years my grandmother spent on this world. At the time of publishing, my mother was 87 years old, and I was doing everything I could to follow in the footsteps of these lovely people.

Speaking of the older generation, kimchi recipes were passed down the matriarchal lineage, and my mother learned how to prepare kimchi by employing her senses—touch, hearing, sight, taste, and smell—from a very young age. I implore you to view food, and kimchi in particular, as a full sensory experience rather than just "fuel" for your body. Many Americans eat quickly and without spending much time analysing their meal, which can lead to bloating, cramping, and indigestion. I urge you to take the time to enjoy eating kimchi in a more relaxed manner. In addition to making your meal more enjoyable, eating it slowly also encourages you to eat less overall and allows your body more time to digest it. You will be rewarded if you take the time to appreciate it visually, including all of its tastes, smells, colours, and textures.

The freshness of the cabbage is assessed through touch. My mother instructed me to make sure the slick layer was removed from each napa leaf as I washed the vegetables. It had to "sound" clean, according to my mother: "sak, sak." Food transmission of parasites was simple fifty years ago, making food cleanliness doubly critical. My mother stated you can tell when something is clean by the sound. The water used to wash the cabbage should be "sak sak" clean.

My halmeoni told my mother that the colour combinations of green, red, white, and yellow in particular were crucial for our minds and appetites when consuming kimchi. Garlic shoots, green onions, and red pepper flakes all contribute to the dish's vibrant crimson colour. My favourite colour pairing of cabbage and radish was white, while ginger and garlic were best represented by the light and fragrant colour yellow. Kimchi is made with essential ingredients including ginger and garlic. They not only possess long-used therapeutic qualities, but they also contain the natural bacteria required to facilitate fermentation. I often tell people, "You can always make kimchi as long as you have ginger, garlic, sea salt, and a vegetable." Everything else is a bonus and simply enhances the dish's flavours and aesthetic appeal.

What You Need: The Fundamentals

It's crucial to understand everything you'll need and the steps involved in producing kimchi before we get started. Fortunately, it's really simple and doesn't take much time, so the rewards in terms of improved health are definitely worth the effort.

First, keep in mind the fundamental kitchenware listed in Chapter 3:

- Clean Knife

- chopping block

- a large mixing bowl

- Colander

- Grater for fruit

- (To handle the red pepper flakes) Gloves

- Mason jars or other sealed glass jars

- Earthenware jars (optional; you can use glass instead)

Before you go grocery shopping, you should double-check the recipe you use every week. For instance, you'll be preparing Cucumber Kimchi in Week 1 of The Kimchi DietTM, so add cucumbers to your grocery list. However, there are a few components that are necessary in almost all kimchi recipes and that you should keep on hand every week. As follows:

- Vegetables

- Salt from the sun

- Garlic

- Ginger

- The colour green

- Fuji Apple or an Asian Pear

- Finely ground red pepper (optional but very healthy)

Special Ingredients

Four components in particular deserve attention since they are so crucial: sun sea salt, red pepper flakes, garlic, and ginger.

They are what I refer to as "superstar ingredients" because they both enhance the flavour of kimchi and each one offers unique practical superpowers! So let's briefly discuss the advantages of these superstars before continuing.

Salt from the sun

In comparison to other varieties of salt, solar sea salt offers far higher quantities of healthy minerals like magnesium, calcium, and potassium since it is created naturally by solar evaporation in salt pans. Please be aware that purchasing sun sea salt is crucial for the quality and flavour of your kimchi as well as the growth of lactic acid bacteria. According to sensory studies, using refined salt or table salt will cause the texture and crunchiness of the kimchi to be less than ideal. Additionally, some sea salts are inherently deficient in other beneficial minerals and high in sodium chloride. Making kimchi with table salt, which can be iodine-fortified, is not something I can imagine. I wouldn't eat the kimchi that was prepared with it. I could be partial, but I like Korean sea salt. Despite the negative connotations associated with salt, a high-salt diet helps to raise the salt levels in the skin, which increases protection from hazardous microbial infections.[1] As was discussed in Chapter 2, the potassium in kimchi may also reduce the dangers of high blood pressure, which can occasionally result from a diet high in salt.

It's advisable to avoid iodine-enriched salts (such as common table salts), as they can interfere with thyroid function. Brining and fermenting using regular table salt will soften and mash the kimchi vegetables. The crisp texture produced by the osmolarity brining effects is one of the characteristics of good kimchi. Regular table salt may also shorten the preservation time of the kimchi. Instead of lasting three to five months, the kimchi may rot after a few weeks. Mineral content is also essential for bacterial growth.

Finally, certain coarse sea salts have not had the extra bitterns (bitter byproduct of salt manufacture) removed, resulting in bitter taste kimchi. As a result, I recommend purchasing a few to discover which one produces the finest taste kimchi. My family has used Korean sun sea salt from Sinan Bay, South Korea, for generations because it is known for its quality, research, and production practises. It is one of the world's top five tidal flats. It's also Kosher certified and meticulously prepared using a natural drying procedure in a clean seaside environment to generate extremely alkaline salt. It is naturally high in critical minerals and has a superior taste that is free of bitterness. Some of this salt has been roasted at 800 degrees, rendering it pesticide, heavy metal, and radioactive waste product free. However, these versions are more expensive.

If you can't get Korean solar sea salt, coarse, white Celtic sea salt is a good substitute.

Korean Red Pepper Powder, coarse

Three hundred years ago, red pepper was added into kimchi preparation practises to give kimchi a fiery, sweet, and smokey aromatic flavour. The primary element in red peppers, capsaicin, is what gives them their functional and therapeutic characteristics. According to research, capsaicin enhances thermogenesis, which produces an increase in metabolism and energy expenditure, potentially aiding those who are obese.[2] Red pepper contains antioxidants in the form of flavonoids, phenolic acids, carotenoids, vitamin A, ascorbic acid (vitamin C), and tocopherols.[3] As previously said, antioxidants aid in the battle against free radicals, which are connected to ageing and a variety of ailments. Furthermore, red pepper powder has a significant effect on the growth of LAB (lactic acid bacteria) in kimchi, such as the strain

Weissella cibaria,[4], so if you can tolerate a little heat, I highly recommend it for optimum probiotic benefit.

The amount of red pepper powder used in each recipe is determined by the level of spiciness desired, the coarseness of the powder, and the type of kimchi being made. If you add too much salt while making the kimchi paste, you'll get additional bitter overtones. The kimchi will also take longer to ferment, affecting the kimchi microbiome's proper growth. Red pepper, as discovered by Korean scientists in 2013, plays a crucial role in extending the life of kimchi by delaying the fermentation process.

[5] Adding red pepper powder to your kimchi helps extend its shelf life, so don't be scared to use it! You can produce milder kimchi by reducing the amount of red pepper, but keep in mind that the fermentation time will be shorter, and the kimchi will need to be consumed sooner. Also, without the red pepper, you may feel compelled to devour far more kimchi than your stomach can manage, so be careful not to overdo it!

When purchasing Korean red pepper powder, consider the colour as well as the coarseness of the flakes. The colour should be crimson with a touch of dark orange. If the powder is more orange in colour, like a pumpkin, it has likely oxidised after resting on the shelf for some time. If the red pepper powder is an extremely dark red, like a maroon, it will turn your kimchi gloomy and unappealing. When it comes to the coarseness of the red pepper powder, seek for one with flake sizes that are around two millimetres in diameter. If it's ground to a fine powder, like paprika, it will oxidise faster and the paste consistency will be more like mud.

Finally, choose coarse red pepper powder grown in South Korea rather than China. Despite the significant price difference, you'll love the level of purity in the Korean edition. Look for "Product of Korea" or "Origin: Korea" on the package label, rather than "P.R.O.C.", "Origin: China", "Chine", or "Product of China."

Garlic

Korea consumes the most garlic per capita of any country in the planet. In fact, I've never cooked kimchi without fresh garlic, or manuel. My mother claims that as long as you have salt and garlic, you can make any type of kimchi. Ginger, red pepper, and pear provide flavour to kimchi, although they are not required ingredients in the same way that garlic is.

Garlic includes a variety of therapeutic chemicals, including allicin, which is considered to be a powerful antioxidant.[6] It also aids in the reduction of LDL cholesterol[7] and has antimicrobial characteristics.

According to Arzanlou's 2016 study, the allicin molecule found in garlic has an inhibiting effect on the actions and life-cycle of strep bacteria, making it a highly useful ally for human immune system.[8] Garlic has long been touted as an immune booster. One study indicated that participants who took one garlic pill daily for four months had fewer viral infections and recovered faster than those who took a placebo.[9] Garlic is not only an all-around superfood with several health advantages; it also plays a significant role in the growth of lactic acid bacteria in kimchi.

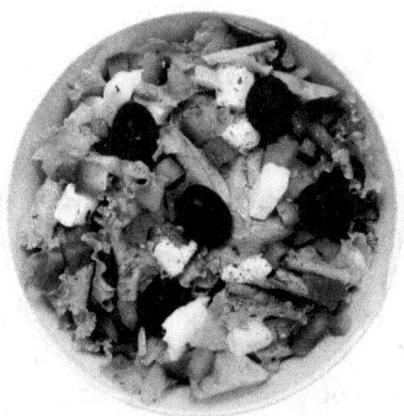

One incredible story I still hear from my mother is about how garlic saved her girlfriend's life during the Korean

War. My mother had to flee south from Inchon with her girl-friend's family when she was about eighteen years old. During the perilous trek, her acquaintance developed cholera, a terrible intestinal bacterial infection that killed the majority of people back then. Her buddy was on the verge of death when her friend's mother crushed two bulbs of fresh garlic, mixed it with rice porridge, and served it to her every day for a week. She gradually began to improve. Her cholera symptoms and dysentery were fully treated after a few weeks on this garlic regimen. Koreans appreciate garlic's therapeutic properties and use it in a variety of dishes, including, of course, kimchi!

Ginger

Ginger is a root of the Zingiber officinale plant that has been used for generations in traditional Korean and Chinese herbal medicine to treat nausea and vomiting, pain, digestive issues, and the common cold. It's also a potent decongestant and antihistamine. Many of these beliefs are now supported by research. Gingerols, powerful molecules found in ginger, have been shown to help with nausea, arthritis, and pain relief, as well as having anti-inflammatory, anticancer, antibacterial, and anti-allergenic qualities, as well as being protective against diabetes, heart disease, and liver disease.[10] Ginger can assist with practically everything.

Not only is ginger a tasty lead component in kimchi, but it also has the unique ability to mask the garlic smell. As previously stated, add one-half teaspoon fresh ginger or a quarter teaspoon ginger powder to hot water, swirl it in the mouth, and swallow. A few drinks will get rid of the strong kimchi and garlic odour that some individuals get.

Drinking a cup of ginger tea is the best way to get rid of kimchi breath!

This method also works while washing dishes. To remove the kimchi odour from the glass jars, simply clean them with soap and water before filling them with warm water. To the clean water, add a half teaspoon of ginger powder. Turn it upside down for 24 hours with the lid closed. The lid can also be deodorised this way. You'll be surprised at how clean it smells afterwards!

Another crucial kimchi tip. The garlic-to-ginger ratio in all of my kimchi recipes is 2:1. Use twice the amount of garlic as ginger.

Extra Ingredient

Kimchi can be made using a variety of other delectable herbs, spices, fruits, and vegetables in addition to these "superstar" elements. Some recipes also include:

- Organic Brown Rice Flour

- Sauce with anchovies

- Paste of Salted Shrimp

- Dashima or Kombu (Dried Kelp)

Because the ingredients listed above do not spoil rapidly, you should buy them on your first shopping trip, along with the cucumbers, garlic, ginger, spring onions, sea salt, and red pepper powder.

Making Kimchi in 4 Simple Steps

1. Vegetable Brining and Preparation

2. Sub-ingredient Preparation

3. Combine the Kimchi Paste and the Vegetables

4. Temperature Control and Storage

The First Step: Cleaning and Brining Kimchi

Let's begin with the cleaning and brining. All outstanding kimchi recipes begin with proper hygiene and cleanliness of your equipment. Before you begin, wash your hands, wipe down the counters, and use very clean utensils. They do not, however, need to be sterilised; they simply need to be clean. Avoid using antibacterial soap on your hands. This soap kills both beneficial and dangerous germs. Kimchi does not require a "starter" culture because it obtains the lactic acid bacteria directly from your hands. You are the initiator of culture!

The practise of brining is essential for kimchi fermentation and good lactic acid bacteria growth.

Brining is defined as "a method of soaking a food product in a saturated salt water solution." Nature's disinfectant is salt. Brining eliminates undesired pathogenic bacteria and fungus through osmotic activity, which can reduce the growth of microbial toxin. As the vegetable moves from a low sodium to a high sodium environment, water is pulled out of its cell walls.

The beauty of lactic acid bacteria is that it develops quickly in a salty environment, whereas more pathogenic bacteria struggle. Salt also prepares and "sweats" the veggies, allowing them to bend more freely without breaking at the end of the brining process. This gives kimchi its delightful crunchy texture.

Traditionally, brining and preparation in the process of manufacturing kimchi vary from family to family, much as recipes varied depending on location and availability of seafood and other unique sub-ingredients. The brining duration and amount of salt used will vary depending on the vegetable fermented, as mentioned in the recipes section of Chapter 5.

In general, there are three primary methods for brining vegetables for kimchi:

1. Only Solar Sea Salt

2. Solar Sea Salt Solution of 10% with Water

3. Solar Sea Salt Brining and Sea Salt Solution Combined

All of the kimchi recipes in this book use the first brining process, which solely uses sun sea salt. This approach was chosen for two reasons. For starters, this is how my mother and grandmother taught me, so it has the benefit of old wisdom on its side. Second, you must use tap water to make saline solution (unless you want to use purified water, which is more expensive), and it can be contaminated with toxicants that are harmful to your digestive system and microbiome, such as chlorine, chloramines, fluoride, arsenic, uranium, and other chemicals. It's best to stick to only salt!

Each recipe will include thorough instructions on how to prepare the veggies to be brined, how much solar sea salt to use, and how long to brine the vegetables for each recipe in the recipe section.

The first stage in brining is to wash, trim, cut, and prepare the veggies to be brined.

These veggies are typically used in the preparation of kimchi:

- Cucumbers

- Mustard Sprouts

- Baby Broccoli

- The Korean Radish

- Cabbage Napa

- Daikon

- Turnips

- Tops of beets

- Tops of Radishes

- Onion Green

- Cabbage, Purple or Green

Second, place the prepared vegetables in a glass bowl and equally sprinkle with solar sea salt. Each recipe will specify how much solar sea salt to need in order to brine properly. Cover the bowl and set it aside for many hours.

If you want to give your kimchi a more "umami" flavour while being vegan (fish sauce or prawn paste provide that extra burst of spiciness), adding kelp water to the kimchi recipe is a terrific alternative. Make kelp water throughout the brining process by soaking three to four pieces (3 inches x 3 inches) of dried kelp in a dish of 4 ounces of room temperature filtered water. The kelp will soften gradually in the water, releasing a gentle ocean scent and seaweed extract. This kelp water can be utilised as a substitute for seafood, adding moisture to the kimchi paste. I consider kelp water to be an optional ingredient, and you don't have to include it to every kimchi recipe; it tastes excellent without it as well, but I would love for you to explore with it!

Third, inspect the vegetables to see if they've released enough water to bend without snapping. To give the vegetables that crisp bite, they may need to release more water. If more time is required, distribute the vegetables and season them on all sides. Allow them to "sweat" more. This is the most critical phase, in my opinion, because the length of time and amount of salt used will determine if all pathogenic bacteria have been eradicated. Checking for perfect crunchiness improves flavour and allows you to establish the ideal saline environment for maximal lactic acid bacteria growth.

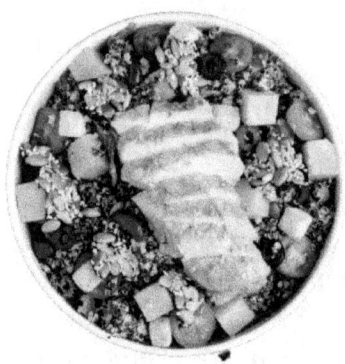

Fourth, once the vegetables have been brined sufficiently, rinse them only once (for the vegan version) by swiftly dipping them into a dish of fresh cold water. If you want to add anchovy fish sauce or salted prawns to your kimchi paste, rapidly immerse the veggies in cool water twice.

Finally, rinse your vegetables in a colander for 15-30 minutes. Taste it- it should be a little salty, but not so much that you want to spit it out. The vegetable should have a crisp texture with minimal water content. Now that the vegetables have been brined, they can be combined with the kimchi paste.

Step 2: Make the Sub-ingredients

So, how exactly do we make the kimchi paste? I'm glad you inquired!
The kimchi ingredients will be washed, trimmed, diced, grated, or julienned. Here is a list of regularly used sub-ingredients, which will change depending on the recipe:Carrot GarlicFish with Ginger Anchovies

- Sauce

- Garlic and ChivesShrimp Salted

- Onions in Green

- Paste

- OnionKelp (Dried)(Optional)
- pears or applesWater from radish kelp)
- Sweet Rice Flour (optional, if making rice porridge)
- (Optional) sugar

I've only mentioned the main sub-ingredients for traditional kimchi, not the ones that are hard to get in conventional grocery shops, like minari (Korean watercress-also known as water dropwort).

If you're vegan, obviously leave out the anchovy fish sauce and salted prawn paste and substitute the seafood with the kelp water described in Step 1 of the brining section, but the taste and quality of the kimchi will suffer as a result. The saltiness of the seafood items helps to kill off nasty bacteria while also adding flavour to the sauce. That is why, if you intend to add the seafood items, I recommend rinsing the brined vegetables twice with cold water. You'll want to keep the brined vegetables saltier without the seafood ingredients by washing them only once with cold water. To prepare 100% plant-based kimchi, salt the veggies more to prevent fungal growth and eradicate pathogenic germs.

Personally, I enjoy both kinds of kimchi, with and without fish. I also enjoy making it the way my forefathers did hundreds of years ago--without the use of any fire, gas or electricity! As a result, I don't add sweet rice flour porridge to my kimchi paste because it requires a heating element to prepare. Koreans enjoy using oatmeal because it improves the consistency of the kimchi paste, adds volume, thickens it, and allows it to readily adhere to the brined veggies. It also feeds the lactic acid bacteria and gives the kimchi a sweeter flavour. My mother makes kimchi with rice porridge, but I discovered that grated pear is a fantastic substitute and have been making kimchi without it for years.

Sugar is a popular ingredient in kimchi, but studies show that the sugar is digested by the lactic acid bacteria and that you aren't taking it as raw, useless calories. Although the sugar and rice porridge aid in the growth of the probiotics, I add grated fruit to bring out the sweet note in the kimchi instead.

Step 3: Combine the Kimchi Paste and the Vegetables

After you've chopped all of the ingredients, combine them in a glass dish and thoroughly combine to form a paste. This is my favourite step; the combination of garlic, ginger, and red pepper makes my mouth swim, and the deep red paste colour is amazing! I also like to taste the kimchi paste before adding it to the brined vegetables to check for flavour.

The paste will be smeared atop the veggies (as with Radish Kimchi), blended into each layer (as with Napa Kimchi), or packed into the vegetable (as with Cucumber Kimchi) depending on the type of kimchi you're creating. After adding the paste to the brined veggies, the kimchi is ready to store and ferment.

The recipe part of the next chapter contains full directions on how to produce the kimchi paste for each recipe.

Step 4: Temperature Regulation and Storage

The final mixture of brined vegetables and kimchi paste must be added to storage jars that do not affect the kimchi's quality or flavour. We also don't want any toxins in the kimchi. Glass canning jars with lids work well for me, and I've gathered a variety of sizes and shapes over the years. Metal and plastic containers leech off residue, making them unsuitable for kimchi storage. Because some of my patients are allergic to nickel, stainless steel containers can be a major issue for them as well. Please don't use plastic.They are harmful to the ecosystem in several ways, and they also include xenoestrogens, which are hormone disruptors that can seep into your food.

It is critical to use the correct jar size. If it's too big and you don't have enough vegetables to fill it up, there will be too much oxygen in the jar, which might lead to fungal development. If you don't give enough space for carbon dioxide gas formation and fermentation, you may have an overflow of kimchi juice after a few days. Allow about an inch to an inch and a half of space at the top of the jar. During the first few days of fermentation, I always leave the kimchi jar in a large bowl in case there is an overflow.

When filling the jar, make sure to pack the vegetables tightly. Fill the jar halfway and squeeze out as much oxygen and bubbles as possible with your fist or a wooden spoon. This extracts the liquid from the vegetables while retaining the paste and juices. Fungi can grow on the exposed surface of the vegetable, where oxygen is readily available. Continue pressing the vegetables down until the jar is full, leaving approximately an inch at the top.

I have read about people's kimchi jars breaking due to fermentation overexpansion. This has never occurred to me since after the initial 24-48 hours of fermentation, I 'burp' the jar by unscrewing the lid halfway and expelling the carbon dioxide gas. You may even buy elaborate fermenting kits with built-in gas releasers in the lids. Due to my kimchi refrigerator, the burping lids make no sense to me. It's deep and broad, so I can stack my bottles on top of each other, saving room. I can have up to thirty jars open at the same time!

Some folks may prefer that the kimchi vegetables and juice do not come into contact with the interior of the jar's lid. If you're worried about this, lay a sheet of parchment paper between the jar and the lid. I don't usually use metal lids since they corrode and discolour the glass jar where the lid contacts it. I also have a couple vintage-style glass jars with wire-bale snap closures that work nicely, but they contain rubber gaskets that can deteriorate over time and need to be replaced. I use parchment paper in these jars since I don't want the scent of rubber in my kimchi.

After filling your jars with veggies, leave them out at room temperature, away from sunshine, for the first fermentation phase before putting them in the refrigerator. Don't forget to put a basin below to catch any spills.

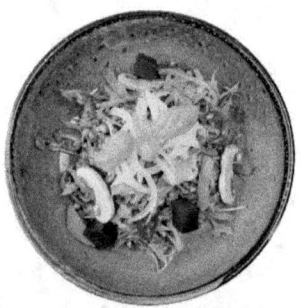

The initial fermentation temperature is crucial since it determines how quickly the kimchi ferments and ripens. In the summer, if the room temperature is above 75 degrees Fahrenheit, I only leave the jar out for 24-36 hours before putting it in the refrigerator, whereas in the winter, if the room temperature is below 68 degrees Fahrenheit or even lower, I may leave the jar out for two or three days to ferment. After 24 hours, taste the kimchi to check how it's progressing. The slower the fermentation and multiplication of lactic acid bacteria, the colder the environment. In a cold environment, Napa cabbage kimchi can take a long time to ferment and may require additional time--four to six days of initial fermentation.

This clever approach allowed Koreans to eat kimchi during the cold. Koreans stopped the brined veggies from freezing over by placing them in clay jars and keeping them underground for insulation, allowing the fermentation to take its time despite the hard winter.

An Introduction to Kimchi Fermentation

After storing your kimchi, the fermentable carbohydrates in the vegetable will be consumed by lactic acid bacteria. The lactic acid bacteria will multiply, eliminate harmful organisms, and further preserve the veggie. As previously stated, lactic acid fermentation is a highly desirable and practical technique of preserving vegetables. It is inexpensive, uses no energy or gas, reduces food waste, and produces a diverse organoleptic experience--a feast for the senses!

The number of organic acids in kimchi grows while the amount of sugar decreases throughout fermentation. The pH falls with the number of days stored at room temperature. Kimchi fermentation is primarily driven by three bacteria genera: Leuconostoc, Lactobacillus, and Weisella. Leuconostoc dominates the early fermentation stage, followed by Lactobacillus and then Weissella, however as fermentation develops, Lactobacillus and Weissella grow more. However, after several weeks of fermentation (Day 23 at 4°C), the populations of Leuconostoc rise while Lactobacillus and Weissella drop.[11] There could be hundreds of distinct strains in each taste of kimchi. Remember that a spoonful of kimchi can contain up to 15 billion CFUs of LAB!

The kimchi lactic acid fermentation process involves three stages.

The pH drops quickly at the start of Phase 1, increasing acidity and carbon dioxide (CO_2) levels. Lactic acid bacteria growth and the removal of unwanted microorganisms begin during this phase. There is also a decrease in natural fermentable sugars (mostly fructose and glucose), as the LAB begins converting fermentable carbohydrates into mannitol. Mannitol adds a delicious sweet taste to kimchi without causing an insulin spike, making it an excellent food for diabetics or anyone with other sugar abnormalities. Within the first five to seven days of fermentation, other end products such as organic acids like lactic acid, acetate, and carbon dioxide are formed.

During Phase 2, the acidity drops continuously, as evidenced by a rapid decline in pH and an increase in CO_2 levels. The effervescent bubbles created while opening a bottle of fermented kimchi demonstrate this. It's incredibly titillating to feel the bubbles in your mouth as you bite into it! From Days 7 to 21, LAB continues to diminish the natural sugars.

The acidity, pH, and CO_2 levels are similar in the final stage of fermentation, Phase 3, and most of the sugars have been utilised and reduced by the lactic acid bacteria. This third phase typically begins on Day 21 and might last for months. Kimchi's shelf life is determined by salinity, season, storage temperature, and the type of vegetable fermented. Cucumber kimchi, for example, should be consumed within three weeks of preparation; otherwise, it will get soggy. However, napa kimchi can be stored in the refrigerator for four to five months and still taste delicious.

Kimchi overripens after months of storage, but don't throw it away! Overripe napa kimchi can be cooked and used to season a variety of foods, including kimchi fried quinoa, kimchi beef stew, kimchi pancakes, kimchi omelettes, and more. I create the traditional kimchi jjigae with overripe kimchi, a stew-like dinner packed of veggies and doenjang, fermented soybean paste.

14 Kimchi Making Suggestions

1. Use sun sea salt from Korea or white Celtic sea salt.

2. Use coarse Korean red pepper powder, not Chinese red pepper powder.

3. Use fresh garlic and ginger rather than powdered garlic and ginger.

4. Fill a glass jar to the top, leaving 1-2 inches for carbon dioxide gas production and the release of surplus water. The lactic acid bacteria develop better when the vegetables are exposed to less oxygen.

5. Be gentle with the ginger. The proportion of garlic to ginger is always 2:1.

6. Vegan kimchi requires more brining time (fish sauce and prawn paste add additional salt to the kimchi paste).

Sugar is optional. Sugar is additional "food" for the growth of lactic acid bacteria, so you won't be consuming it when the kimchi is fully mature. Superfood that is low in calories!

8. Green onions have the ability to make kimchi juice "sticky." There is no need to be concerned; it is safe to consume; but, if it bothers you, substitute chives or garlic chives.

9. Before incorporating the kimchi paste, taste the brined kimchi. It should not be too salty.
10. Having more kimchi paste is preferable to not having enough. The ideal amount of kimchi sauce will influence fermentation pace, yeast overgrowth, and flavour.

11. While filling the jar, push the contents down with a spoon on a regular basis to release as much oxygen as possible and express more liquid out of the veggies.

12 Place a basin beneath the kimchi container in case of overflow during the first several days of fermenting.

13. Don't open the cover during the first few days of fermentation unless you're tasting it to assess how ripe it is before refrigerating. I generally taste it 24 hours later.

14. The refrigerator works best at temperatures ranging from 37 to 41 degrees Fahrenheit (3 to 5 degrees Celsius). If the temperature is too low, the kimchi will take a long time to ripen, and if it is too high, the kimchi will deteriorate.

To get rid of kimchi breath, drink ginger tea. It's also effective as a digestion aid!

Chapter 5: Recipes of Kimchi Diet

These are some of my family's favourite kimchi dishes, and they're ordered in the order that they should be cooked and eaten according to The Kimchi DietTM plan. They've been passed down through numerous generations, they're tried and true, and I present them to you with love. Enjoy!

For your convenience, here is another Quick Summary of The Kimchi DietTM Timeline.

Phase 1: Days 1-14

Day 1: Make Cucumber Kimchi.

Day 3-4: Begin eating 2 to 3 pieces of one cucumber kimchi floret per day.

Day 7-8: Work your way up to eating the complete cucumber kimchi floret on a regular basis.

Day 8: Make kimchi with baby bok choy, mustard greens, radish tops or beetroot tops.

Day 8-14: Continue to eat 1 cucumber kimchi floret every day.

Phase 2: Days 14-28

Day 14-21: Finish the cucumber kimchi and begin eating 1 tablespoon of the Phase 2 kimchi of your choice (baby bok choy, mustard greens, radish tops or beetroot tops). Increase to two tablespoons every day.

Day 21: Make root vegetable kimchi (radish, daikon, turnip or rutabaga).

Day 21-28: Continue eating Phase 2 kimchi.

Phase 3: Days 28-42

Day 28: Finish the Phase 2 kimchi and begin eating one to two teaspoons of the root vegetable kimchi (radish, daikon, turnip or rutabaga).

Day 28: Make the napa cabbage kimchi.

Day 28-42: Continue to consume 2-3 tablespoons of both Phase 2 and Phase 3 kimchi daily.

Phase 4: Days 42-56 and Beyond

Day 42: Consume one to two tablespoons of napa cabbage kimchi and keep an eye out for symptoms.

Day 42-56: Continue eating the leftover Phase 2 and Phase 3 kimchi and introducing napa cabbage kimchi into your diet. Increase your kimchi consumption to 4 tablespoons each day.

4 Steps to Making Kimchi

1. Brining

Wash and trim the main vegetable(s) to be salted and brined for a particular amount of time.

2. Making Kimchi Paste

Wash, trim, dice, grate, or julienne the sub-ingredients.

3. Make the Kimchi Paste

Prepare the paste and combine it with the brined veggies.

4. Storage and Temperature Control

Fill storage jars halfway with the final vegetable mixture and keep at room temperature.

Days 1-14 of Phase 1 Cucumber (Oi) Kimchi

Ingredients

- 8 seedless, waxless Kirby (pickling), Persian, or Lebanese cucumbers or 4 long Korean or English (hot house) cucumbers 2 tbsp coarse solar sea salt

Kimchi Paste Ingredients

- 1 medium carrot, thinly sliced into matchsticks 1 to 12 inch length or shred with a grater if time is short1 cup daikon, finely cut into matchsticks 1-12 inch in length

- 1 cup garlic (Buchu) or ordinary chives, cut into 12-34" inch chunks

- 2 tsp minced garlic

- 1 teaspoon grated ginger

- Half cup grated Asian pear, Fuji apple, or 2 tablespoons rice porridge*

- 2 tablespoons anchovy fish sauce or kelp water (optional)

12 cup Korean red pepper powder* (lower the quantity for milder kimchi)1 tbsp purified water

*If you are sensitive to spicy foods, you can leave out the red pepper powder in all kimchi recipes, but you will have to alter the initial time of fermentation at room temperature by a couple of hours and eat it before it over-ripens. Red pepper powder inhibits the fermentation and ripening process, so adjust

appropriately. If you don't want to add red pepper or seafood, salt the brined vegetable before adding the sub-ingredient kimchi paste.

Instructions Brining time: 1 hour

1. Rinse and drain the cucumbers. Optional: To make kelp water, soak three to four pieces (3 inches × 3 inches) of dried kelp in a cup of 4 ounces of clean water at room temperature.

2. Remove the ends of each cucumber and cut it into 2-3 inch slices. If using Kirby's, cut them in half, or if using longer cucumbers, cut them into three pieces, each about 3 inches long.

3. Place a cucumber piece on the cutting board and cut it down through the diameter of the cucumber vertically (lengthwise), leaving 12 inch on the bottom of each cucumber piece uncut. Then, at a 90-degree angle, cut perpendicularly through the diameter without completely cutting through, forming a "X." This will turn each 3-inch cucumber slice into a 4-petal floret, giving room to add the kimchi sauce after brining.

4. Place the cucumber florets in a large glass or ceramic dish and equally sprinkle the coarse sea salt on the interior and outside of each floret. Allow the bowl to brine for an hour away from sunlight. After 30 minutes, you'll notice some "sweat" water at the bottom of the dish. Toss the cucumber florets a couple of times, then

set aside for 30 minutes to brine. Chop, mince, and grate the materials for the kimchi paste.

5. After brining, the cucumber should be supple and easy to bend without cracking in half. Place the brined cucumber florets in a colander (discard the brined salty liquid) and swiftly dip into a large bowl of fresh water once to remove any excess salt and debris. Drain for 10 minutes in a colander while you create the kimchi paste.

Kimchi Tip: If you intend to use anchovy fish sauce in your kimchi paste, swiftly dip the cucumber twice in the bowl of water. Try not to leave the brined cucumber in the water for too long. Otherwise, too much salt will be taken out of the brined veggies, impairing the fermentation process. This 'double dip' rinse is only necessary if your recipe contains fish sauce or prawn paste.

Making Kimchi Paste

- 1. Combine the garlic, ginger, grated pear, fish sauce or kelp water, and red pepper flakes in a large glass or ceramic bowl. Wear disposable food preparation gloves to protect your skin from the red pepper, and combine the ingredients to make a paste. Mix in the carrots, chives, and daikon to the paste.

- 2. Stuff the chive/carrot kimchi paste into each cucumber floret. As you stuff the next floret, set each packed floret aside in the bowl. Don't worry if the florets break apart; the dish will still taste delicious!

- 3. Apply additional kimchi paste to the outside of the cucumber florets.

Kimchi Tip: It's preferable to have too much paste than not enough; create more if necessary!

Temperature Control and Storage

- 1. I like to bottle many jars per recipe so that while you're eating from one, the others can continue to ferment without being disturbed. The remaining bottles will remain untouched and boiling with carbonation until you are ready to consume them.

Fill the jar halfway with florets, then press the florets down with a wooden spoon to bring the oxygen bubbles to the surface. This will aid in the prevention of yeast growth. Fill to the brim and expel as many oxygen bubbles as possible.

Pushing down on the cucumber florets causes more water to be excreted. This additional juice submerges the cucumber florets, keeping oxygen away from the vegetables and preventing yeast growth. Don't be concerned if you still notice bubbles. More water will be released as it ferments, and bubbles will rise to the surface.

Finally, add one tablespoon of purified water to any remaining kimchi paste in the bowl and evenly divide in each bottle before sealing with a lid.

Close the lid over the parchment paper and place it on top of the jar. If there is an overflow, the kimchi will not come into contact with the plastic or metal cover. Parchment paper also aids in keeping the lid in place.

- 2. Do not totally fill the jar. Allow roughly 1 inch from the top of the rim for clearance. As fermentation progresses, carbon dioxide emissions created by the LAB accumulate, and more water sweats out from the cucumbers, causing the amount of liquid and kimchi to climb to the top. There's a danger the kimchi will overflow if you fill the jar all the way.

Finally, place a plate or basin beneath the container to collect any extra juice that may drip out during the first several days of fermentation. For one or two days, leave the container out in room temperature (68-72 degrees Fahrenheit) away from the sun. Your glass container has a very minimal chance of cracking. To avoid difficulties, 'burp' the kimchi bottle after a few days of fermentation by slowly turning the cap and letting the gas out, much like you would with a bottle of carbonated water. Perform this over the washbasin. The carbon dioxide effect may surprise you!

- 3. Refrigerate at 3-5 degrees Celsius (37-41 degrees Fahrenheit) with a dish underneath to catch any potential overflow.

- 4. Follow the instructions in Chapter 3 of Phase 1 of The Kimchi DietTM.

Note: I prefer to sample the fermented kimchi right before putting it in the fridge.

First and foremost, I want to taste the kimchi. I'm seeking for a flavour that is slightly salty, sweet, tangy, and savoury. Second, the flavour indicates the rate of fermentation, which dictates how soon I must consume it before it overripens. If I think it needs more time to ferment, I'll leave it out at room temperature for another 6-8 hours.

The amount of salt used during the brining process, as well as the temperature of the ambient area where the jars will be housed throughout the first fermentation process, all influence the rate of fermentation. Kimchi ferments more slowly in the winter. It will ferment faster in the summer. The slower the kimchi ferments, the saltier it is. Finally, if you use red pepper powder, the kimchi will ferment more slowly. All of these variations will become apparent as you prepare kimchi from season to season.

What I like about cucumber kimchi is that it can be eaten immediately after it's made. This also allows anyone who has had a lot of digestive troubles to gently integrate kimchi into their diet without any significant reactions, allowing them to gradually build up a healthier microbiome. The LAB in the kimchi expands exponentially with each day of fermentation, and if you eat little portions daily, you'll reap the benefits--and in no time, you'll be transforming your inflamed, dysbiotic gut into one with a rich, diverse, and balanced microbiome!
Cucumber kimchi should be consumed within two weeks, but the liquid should be saved! It still contains a lot of probiotics and postbiotics (LAB metabolites). You can consume a couple of teaspoons every day to continue on your path to bright health.
Recipe for Phase 2: Days 14-28

Kimchi with Baby Bok Choy, Mustard Greens (Gat), Radish Tops or Beet Tops

Ingredients

- 1 pound baby bok choy, mustard greens, radish tops or beet greens

- 1 tbsp solar sea salt, coarse

Ingredients for Kimchi Paste

- 2 green onion stalks, cut into 1-inch chunks

- Half cup Korean radish or daikon, thinly sliced into 1-1 12 inch matchsticks

- 1 tsp. minced garlic

- Half teaspoon ginger, grated

- 1/4 cup grated Asian pear, Fuji apple, or rice porridge*

- 2 tbsp (optional) Korean red pepper powder

- 1 tablespoon optional fish sauce or kelp water

- 1 tbsp. filtered water

Instructions Time to brine: 1-2 hours

- 1. Thoroughly soak and rinse the bok choy leaves, mustard greens, radish tops and beetroot tops. Remove the stem's base and peel off each leaf. Drain through a colander.

- 2. Place the rinsed green veggies in a big glass or ceramic bowl and sprinkle with solar salt. Increase the "sweating," sucking out extra water from the thicker area of the leaf, by adding more salt to the stems and going lighter on the soft leaves.

- 3. Cover the basin and brine the bok choy for up to 2 hours. The brining time for mustard greens, radish and beetroot tops will be less than an hour.

- 4. Turn the leaves over halfway through the brining procedure. You'll notice some water at the bottom of the dish. Prepare the kimchi paste components 30 minutes before the brining is finished by chopping, mincing, and grating the sub-ingredients.

- 5. The bok choy or greens will be deeper in colour and more flexible at the end of the brining process. Place the brined veggies in a strainer (discard the brined salty liquid) and swiftly dip the greens into a big bowl of fresh water once to remove any excess salt and debris. Shake off excess water and drain for 10 minutes in a colander while you make the kimchi paste.

Kimchi Tip: If you're going to add fish sauce to your kimchi paste, don't forget to double dip it!

Kimchi Sauce

- 1. Combine the garlic, ginger, grated pear, red pepper flakes, and fish sauce or kelp water in a large glass or ceramic bowl. Put on disposable food preparation gloves and combine the ingredients to make a paste. Mix in the green onion and daikon to the paste.

- 2. Stir in the brined bok choy or greens, coating each leaf thoroughly with the kimchi paste

Temperature Control and Storage

- 1. Store the cucumber kimchi in the same manner as described in the cucumber kimchi recipe. I normally use glass bottles that are 16 or 32 ounces in size. Fill the glass container halfway with greens and press down with a wooden spoon to raise the oxygen bubbles and squeeze out excess liquid, allowing it to rise to the surface and submerge the greens.

- 2. Continue to fill until the container is full, forcing as many oxygen bubbles out as possible. After that, add 1 tablespoon of purified water to any leftover kimchi paste in the dish and evenly distribute it into each container. Before covering with a lid, leave about 1 inch of room at the top of the rim. You can also line the lid with parchment paper before closing it.

- 3. Leave the kimchi bottles at room temperature (68-72 degrees Fahrenheit) for 24 hours, away from the sun. Don't forget to place a dish beneath the bottle to catch any juice spills.

- 4. After 24 hours of fermentation, "burp" each bottle and taste it, as described in the Cucumber Kimchi recipe.

- 5. Place in the refrigerator at 37-41 degrees Fahrenheit (3-5 degrees Celsius) with a dish underneath to catch any probable overflow.

- 6. Follow the instructions in Chapter 3 of Phase 2 of The Kimchi DietTM.

Days 28-42, Phase 3 Recipe: Radish (Kkakdugi) Kimchi

Ingredients

- 2 lbs. Korean radish, daikon, turnip, or rutabagas

- 2 tbsp solar sea salt, coarse

Ingredients for Kimchi Paste

- 2 tablespoons garlic mince

- 1 teaspoon ginger, grated

- 1/4 cup garlic or chives, cut into 12-34" inch chunks

- 1/2 cup grated Asian pear, Fuji apple, or other apple

- 2 teaspoons rice porridge*

- 1/2 cup Korean red pepper powder (less for a milder flavour)

- Optional: 1 teaspoon minced salted prawns, fish sauce or kelp water1 tbsp. filtered water

Instructions Brining time: 1hour 30 minutes-2 hours

1. Rinse, clean, and remove any bruises or lodged filth. Peel the skin off with a potato peeler. As long as the peel is clean, you can leave it on. Cut the radish into 1 1/2 X 4-inch segments lengthwise and place in a large glass or ceramic basin. Optional: Soak three to four pieces (3 inches × 3 inches) of dried kelp in a bowl of 4 ounces of filtered water at room temperature to make kelp water. Set aside, covered.

2. Evenly sprinkle the sea salt over the cubed radish. Cover and leave to brine for 1 12-2 hours away from direct sunlight.

3. Water will have been released from the radish cubes and will be sitting at the bottom of the basin halfway through the brining procedure. Toss the radish cubes and set aside for the remaining brining time.

4. The radish cubes will have more "give" at the end of the brining procedure. Place the brined radish in a colander (discard the brined salty liquid) and immediately rinse with fresh water to remove any excess salt or dirt. Drain for 10 minutes in a colander while you make the kimchi paste.

If you're going to add fish sauce to your kimchi paste, don't forget to double dip!

Kimchi Sauce

1. Combine the garlic, ginger, grated pear, red pepper flakes, minced salted prawns, fish sauce or kelp water in a large glass or ceramic bowl. Put on disposable food preparation gloves and combine the ingredients to make a paste. Mix in the green chives into the paste.

2. Toss the drained, brined radish cubes with the kimchi paste, coating them evenly.

Temperature Control and Storage

1. Store the cucumber kimchi in the same manner as described in the cucumber kimchi recipe. Fill the glass jar halfway with brined and seasoned radish and press down with a wooden spoon to release the oxygen bubbles. This will cause extra liquid to rise to the surface, drowning the radish.

Don't be concerned if you don't see any more liquid. More water will "sweat" out during the fermentation process, increasing the volume of kimchi juice.

2. Continue to fill to the top while pushing out as many oxygen bubbles as possible. Then, add 1 tablespoon of filtered water to the remaining kimchi paste in the bowl and equally spread it into each container. Before covering with a lid, leave about 1 inch of room at the top of the rim. If desired, add the parchment paper before closing the lid. Place a plate below to catch any kimchi liquid that may overflow.

3. Leave the kimchi bottles at room temperature for 2-3 days, away from the sun, then "burp" each bottle after a few days of fermentation, as indicated in the Cucumber Kimchi recipe. Before refrigerating, conduct a taste test.

4. Place in the refrigerator at 37-41 degrees Fahrenheit (3-5 degrees Celsius) with a dish underneath to catch any probable overflow.

5. Follow the instructions in Phase 3 of The Kimchi DietTM.

Radish kimchi keeps better than other kimchi and can be stored in the refrigerator for months. The kimchi juice is really wonderful, especially after fermenting for 4-6 weeks. I've drizzled it over eggs, vegetables, and even quinoa to add flavour to my meals. I've also used radish juice for fiery Tabasco sauce in my Virgin Bloody Mary drinks, and it tastes fantastic! The recipe is available in the Resource section.

Recipe for Phase 4: Days 42-56 Kimchi with Napa Cabbage (Baechu)

Ingredients

- 1 Napa cabbage, large

- 1/2 cup fine solar sea salt

Ingredients for Kimchi Paste

- 12 cup Korean radish or daikon, thinly sliced into 1-1 12 inch matchsticks

- 2 tablespoons garlic mince

- 1 teaspoon ginger, grated

- 1/4 cup garlic or chives, cut into 12-34" inch chunks12 cup grated Asian pear, Fuji apple, or rice porridge*

- 1/2 cup powdered Korean red pepper

- Optional: 2 teaspoons anchovy fish sauce, prawn paste or kelp water2 tbsp. distilled water

Instructions Time to Brin: 4 hours

1. Halve the cabbage lengthwise. Then chop it again to get four quartered cabbage pieces. All of the leaves should be held in place by the stalk. Remove and discard any wilted or damaged leaves, then thoroughly rinse the remaining leaves under cold running water, especially around the stem. The stem will seem slick at first, but as you brush your thumb over it multiple times, you will notice a "sak sak" clean sound beneath flowing water. Wash all four cabbage pieces thoroughly and drain upside down in a strainer.

2. Place one drained cabbage quarter in a large glass or ceramic bowl, with the leaves facing up. Sprinkle the coarse sea salt evenly throughout each leaf, beginning with the bottom leaf and working your way up, concentrating on the thicker area of each leaf closest to the stem. For the entire napa cabbage, use up to 12 cup of sea salt.

3. Tightly fold the cabbage leaves together and place in a big glass or ceramic bowl, with the inside of the cabbage facing up, to keep the salt tightly tied inside the cabbage leaves. To hold the cabbage leaves closed, place a heavy dish on top. Cover and set aside at room temperature for 4 hours, away from the sun.

4. Check on the cabbage after a couple of hours of brining. Due to the "sweating" induced by the salt

draining the water content out of the leaves, the stem will seem shinier, the leaves brighter in colour, and notably smaller in size. The leaves will be sufficiently flexible to allow the stem to bend without breaking. This will give the kimchi a nice texture and crunch. Extra water will accumulate at the bottom of the bowl; do not discard it. Turn the cabbage over and leave it for a couple of hours more. This, again, is dependent on how salty you like your kimchi.

Optional: Soak three to four pieces (3 inches × 3 inches) of dried kelp in a bowl of 4 ounces of filtered water at room temperature to make kelp water. Set aside, covered.

Prepare the kimchi paste components 30 minutes before the brining is finished by chopping, mincing, and grating the sub-ingredients.

5. Place the brined cabbage in a colander (discard the brined salty liquid) and immediately rinse with cold water to remove any excess salt or debris. I like to taste the brined Napa cabbage at this point. It should have a crisp texture and taste salty like the ocean. You can rinse it one more time if it's too salty.

Kimchi Tip: If you're going to add fish sauce to your kimchi paste, don't forget to double dip it!

6. Gently squeeze out the water and drain it in a colander for 15 minutes while you make the kimchi paste. Kimchi Sauce

1. Combine the garlic, ginger, grated pear, red pepper flakes and anchovy fish sauce, prawn paste or kelp water in a large glass or ceramic bowl. Put on disposable food preparation gloves and combine the ingredients to make a paste. Mix in the green chives and daikon to the paste.

2. Remove one large outside brined leaf from each half of the cabbage and keep aside for later use.

3. Before adding the kimchi paste to the brined cabbage, you can either cut it up into bite-size pieces and then add the kimchi paste, making it easier to eat after fermentation-or you can add the kimchi paste to the cabbage with the leaves attached to the stem, letting it ferment, and then cutting it up each time you want to eat some.

Personally, I like it both ways, but traditionally, Koreans believe that cutting up the kimchi as it's going to be presented to their guests is more honourable and visually pleasing.

4. Here are the two versions: Quick version (Mak Kimchi)

Add the brined cabbage to the large glass bowl of kimchi paste in small, bite-sized 1-2 square inch pieces.

Mix the kimchi paste into the brined cabbage thoroughly while using disposable food preparation gloves. It's now time to put it in the glass containers.

Traditional (Baechu Kimchi) variant

Wearing protective gloves, add the quartered brined cabbage to the large bowl of kimchi paste. Peel back all of the leaves down to the last layer, with the inside of the leaves facing up, and smear the paste onto each leaf.

Add more at the stem of each leaf, where it requires more seasoning. Repeat for each leaf layer.

Once all of the layers have been seasoned, tightly wrap the outer layers of leaves around the inner ones to keep the paste within. Set aside gently so it doesn't unravel, then repeat with the remaining brined cabbage. There should be enough kimchi paste to season each of the brined cabbage quarters. It's now time to put it in the glass containers.

Temperature Control and Storage

1. To prepare kimchi from one full Napa cabbage, use two 16-ounce bottles or one 32-ounce bottle.

2. Follow the same basic storage directions as the Cucumber Kimchi recipe for both variations. Fill the glass container halfway with the seasoned Napa

cabbage and press down with a wooden spoon to force the oxygen bubbles to the surface. This will force extra liquid to the surface, drowning the cabbage.

In a 32-ounce bottle, combine all four wrapped cabbage pieces for the traditional version. The conventional approach is more difficult to extract the gas bubbles without breaking apart the cabbage ball.

3. Add 2 tablespoons of filtered water to any remaining kimchi paste in the dish and evenly spread it into the bottle(s).

4. Leave about 1 inch of space over the rim. Add a single layer of brined cabbage to the top of the seasoned cabbage before covering the lid. This is the one reserved in Step 2 of the Kimchi Paste section. This will look like a "toupee" on top of the seasoned cabbage and will keep oxygen from coming into contact with it throughout the fermentation process, decreasing yeast development.

5. If you like, you can add the parchment paper before sealing the lid. Place a bowl beneath the bottles to catch any spilled kimchi liquid. Leave the kimchi bottles at room temperature for two days, away from the sun, and "burp" each bottle every day. Before refrigerating, conduct a taste test.
6. Refrigerate at 37-41 degrees Fahrenheit (3-5 degrees Celsius) with a dish underneath to collect any potential overflow.

7. Follow the directions in Phase 4 of The Kimchi DietTM.

How to Make Rice Porridge

Ingredients

- 2 tbsp sweet rice flour, organic

- 1 cup distilled water

- 1 cup of purified water and 2 teaspoons of organic sweet rice flour should be combined in a small pot. Bring to a boil, stirring constantly. It will thicken to the consistency of porridge. Place the rice porridge in a bowl to chill while you prepare the kimchi ingredients and paste.

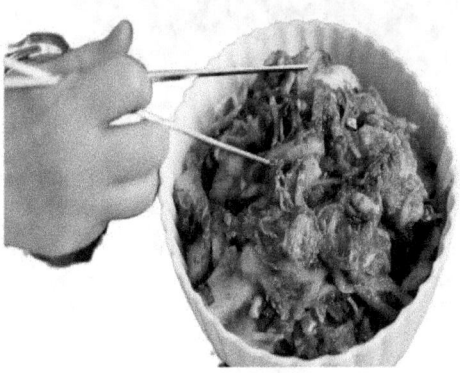

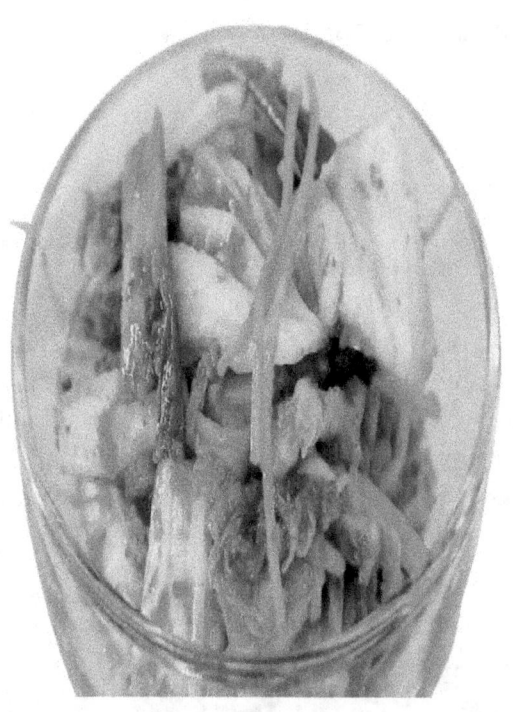